The
ANNAPOLIS
DIET

The
ANNAPOLIS
DIET

Karen Gibson

ST. MARTIN'S PRESS
New York

To the midshipmen who participated in the Naval Academy diet program, the galley cooks, and the Food Service Division of the United States Naval Academy.

My grateful thanks,
Karen

Library of Congress Cataloging in Publication Data

Gibson, Karen.
    The Annapolis diet.

    1. Low-calorie diet—Recipes.   2. Cookery
(Melons)—Recipes.   I. Title.
RM222.2.N44   1985   613.2′5   84-24798
ISBN 0-312-03842-9

First Edition

10 9 8 7 6 5 4 3 2 1

Contents

Acknowledgments

A special thanks to the following people, without whose assistance this book would not have been possible: Food Service Manager Richard P. La Rochelle; Thomas Simmons; Prudente Baysic; Lieutenant Alden Salcedo; Ensign Frazer Frantz; Chief Revacato Luistro; Petty Officer Gerald Ross; Red Romo of the Naval Academy Athletic Department; Commander Trudy Verring, R.N., of the Naval Academy Medical Clinic; Stephanie Rodi, Dietitian; Susan Marlin, R.N.; Douglas Sobel, M.D.; and to all the midshipmen who spent hours on the calorie calculations. Also to my medical advisor, Doctor Herbert J. Mavins III; Elizabeth Johnson, who guided me through the beginning stages of this book and kept me writing; and to Jamey Gibson and Courtney Neeb, who helped me put it on the word processor.

A big thanks to our galley cooks—Lawrence Harris, Shirley Burgess, Kathleen Christ, Ethel Jackson, and Alice Butler—who cooked this diet food perfectly each day for four years.

My thanks also to the Commandant of Midshipmen, Commodore Leon Edney, and Deputy Commandant of Midshipmen, Captain Alfred L. Chearuc, who carefully monitored the diet program and gave me their complete support.

Finally, there just aren't words to express my gratitude to Vice Admiral and Mrs. Edwin C. Waller, who helped test these recipes by dieting along with the midshipmen.

And hats off to the midshipmen who participated in the program and kept the spirit going. Your efforts deserve a "Well done!"

Introduction

I have found a secret weapon for battling excess weight—
melon. During the more than three years I spent at the
United States Naval Academy developing the Annapolis Diet,
I discovered that serving cantaloupe, honeydew, casaba, and
watermelon to the dieting midshipmen helped them lose
weight easily and quickly. One serving of melon was used at
every meal. The midshipmen participating in the program
soon found out that if it was food, "Mrs. Food" (that's my
nickname in the Brigade of Midshipmen) would put melon
in it. I added the melon to help satisfy the sweet tooth. But it
has much more than that to offer. It's refreshing, natural,
low in calories, and filling. Not only that—it's loaded with
vitamin A. All this wrapped up into one delicious sphere!
What's more, as time went by and more and more melon was
served, our midshipmen dieters just couldn't get enough of
it. The mids would come into our diet dining room and ask
immediately what the melon recipe for the meal was. The
simple melon held their interest; it was something to look
forward to.

Cantaloupe was by far the favorite of the dieters. When
compared with that popular diet fruit, grapefruit, the cantaloupe wins hands down. It tastes better, and because it has
fewer calories per ounce, you can eat a larger quantity,
satisfying your hunger pains without jeopardizing your diet.
It's available year round and is usually very reasonably
priced—assets that make it appealing to dieters everywhere.

Would you believe that on the Annapolis Diet you can eat chicken Cacciatore, baked potatoes, lobster Thermidor, beef Stroganoff, spaghetti, and bread and lose 12 pounds in two weeks? The diet was designed for men and women of all ages who love food. I'm over forty and this is the diet that finally helped me lose 30 pounds. I had never before dieted successfully because I just couldn't bear the thought of eating cottage cheese and grapefruit.

Food has been my passion and my profession for the past fifteen years. I've written cookbooks, directed a cooking school, toured the United States giving cooking classes, cooked on television for thousands of viewers, and worked as consulting chef to major food service institutions. I was working as consulting chef and food service advisor to the Naval Academy when the commandant of midshipmen asked the food service officer at the Academy to devise a diet plan for midshipmen who were overweight by navy standards. I was asked to develop such a plan. The Annapolis Diet was the result.

King Hall, the midshipmen's dining area, is a giant room seating 4,500 midshipmen. Delicious entrées typical of American cuisine are served there, each containing over 6,000 calories. Thus, I knew that I had to create menus that were not only nutritious but delicious, satisfying, and appealing to men and women with high expectations. I wanted the food to taste like regular home-cooked meals. It had to dazzle the dieters. I know I was successful because they constantly exclaimed, "This doesn't taste like diet food. It's like mom's cooking." When one midshipman was told that he could go off the diet program because in three and a half weeks he had lost his 20 pounds, he said, "Please don't make me go; I love this food."

The Annapolis Diet contains both menus and gourmet recipes. I often cooked sixteen hours a day while testing these recipes. I was devising the first diet plan ever to be used in the Academy's 137 years of existence, and I knew from the first week that it was successful because the fifteen original dieting midshipmen had lost a total of 117 pounds. All the people who subsequently followed this diet have lost at least 7 pounds the first week and 5 pounds the second week. With those initial 12 pounds gone so fast, the remaining weeks on the diet were easy. All this weight loss was accomplished by *eating*. The dieters were never hungry.

Word traveled fast that something special was going on in the diet kitchen and I had many requests for copies of the recipes. I had the full support of the superintendent of the Naval Academy, the commandant of midshipmen. Medical doctors, dietitians, nurses, and nutritionists checked each recipe and menu to be sure that the daily requirements for nutrition were met. Although I am not a nutritionist, my background in nursing helped me immensely in selecting menus, and my years of teaching food preparation and working with chefs from around the world whose claim to fame was diet food preparation helped to give the Annapolis Diet its variety.

We are living in an era of fads and fallacies. It is a time when those considered good-looking and successful are thin and when fat is seen as not only ugly but bad. I've fought being overweight for ten years. I was 30 pounds overweight and when I looked in the mirror, all I could see were the puffy cheeks of a baby whale. (This may sound irreverent, but it is important to be able to laugh at yourself. Laughter is vital in life but twice as vital while dieting.) Thus I found that the only way to fight obesity is to look at yourself honestly in a full-length mirror. If you don't like what's looking back at you, then ask yourself, "How did I let this happen to me and what can I do to correct it?" I sought to impress this lesson upon my dieters the first day. The day our program started I met the midshipmen in a special dining area. They weighed themselves, and we sat down to enjoy our first breakfast together. I told them: "The body you are in belongs to you.

What you do with it in the next six weeks during this dieting period is up to you." I recited the fat person's classic excuse: "I'm so tall and I have such large bones." All heads nodded in agreement. They knew very well how easy it was to make those constant excuses so that they could eat all their favorite foods. I promised the midshipmen the perfect diet, one that would allow them to eat what they wanted but controlled the amount they ate.

I explained to the midshipmen that the six short weeks they would spend on the diet were a small part of their lives. You, too, will find the six weeks passing quickly, and once you learn how much to eat to maintain your new low weight, you can be free of fighting fat for the rest of your life. The Law of Thermodynamics will prevail. A calorie is a measure of heat and losing weight a matter of very simple mathematics. Anybody who eats less than 11 calories per day per pound of body weight will lose weight. Conversely, if you overeat by one carrot (about 30 calories) each day, in ten years you will have gained 30 pounds. This explanation brought the subject home very fast to the midshipmen, engineering students who were used to working with numbers.

The midshipmen were shocked to hear that the 70 billion or so fat cells filling their uniforms to capacity never die. Fat cells just shrivel up and hang in clusters waiting to be fed a rich dessert, which they can gobble up and store somewhere around the waist or hips. When the brain says celery and the fat cells scream cheesecake, there's no contest. The fat cells will win, and unless you get your eating habits under control you will be overweight forever.

The recipes in this book are quite different, and some may at first appear strange, but stick with them. You will be rewarded in the end. Remember, though, that it isn't wise to cut your calories under 900 per day because you may start losing muscle and you are on this diet to lose fat only. My advice is to talk to your doctor before you start this diet.

Now let's get started!

1

The Rules for Eating

"**G**ood morning, midshipmen," I said to the fifteen nervous uniformed men and women sitting around the table. It was 6:15 A.M. and it was our first meeting. You should have seen their sleepy faces. The one place in the world they did not want to be at that hour was in the special Diet Room having a battleaxe like me telling them that because they had spent too much time at the hamburger shop, I was now going to deprive them of the things they loved the most—french fries, milk shakes, pizza, chili dogs, potato chips, colas. . . !

"First of all, ladies and gentlemen, welcome to the Diet Room, where from this moment forward you are on the melon diet." Fifteen pairs of eyes rolled around in their sockets with a look that said, "Oh, my God! What's next?" The consensus of this group of young people was that Mrs. Food was going to take away their goodies, and they were preparing to be miserable for the next six weeks. Or perhaps I should say starved.

"You have eaten your way to this spot at the table and you are now going to *eat* to get out of here," I continued. "You'll have between 900 and 1,200 calories a day." The chairs rustled as they fidgeted nervously with their last cup of morning coffee. "You will be on this diet for approximately six weeks. Some of you will lose your weight in less time." I could see they were relaxing now. Of course every one of them knew that he or she would be a short-timer. "Meanwhile, you will get your fill of waffles, pancakes, syrup, steak, tacos, shrimp, even lobster." I went on to announce that part of the diet plan included going to a fast food restaurant, and they looked at me in disbelief. I had them now. Maybe they weren't going to starve after all.

"The secret to this diet is melon. You will eat one portion at each meal, and I expect you to eat all of the food that is put in front of you. To make you lose faster, there will be no skipping of meals or cheating on this diet."

"M'am, I don't like onions, green peppers, tomatoes, or spices. Does this food we have to eat contain that stuff?" asked a handsome midshipman who looked like Robert Redford with a body the size of Rosie Greer. Actually, he was the star of the navy's football team. "Midshipman, you'll learn to love them."

This diet is designed to help you lose weight gradually. The goal is to lose 20 pounds and keep it off for the rest of your life. If you allow yourself to gain a few pounds on vacation, on a special weekend, or during all those holiday parties, you can always go back on the plan and take off those extra pounds quickly before they once again become a serious problem. On this diet you must follow nine easy rules for eating everyday.

RULES FOR EATING
1. Eat three meals a day.
2. Eat only when sitting down.
3. Weigh yourself every morning and keep a weight chart.
4. Eat at the same time everyday.
5. Eat slowly.
6. No caffeine.

7. Take one multivitamin per day.

8. Drink eight glasses of water per day and no more than two diet sodas per day.

9. Do not salt your food at the table.

Do these rules seem impossible to follow? They really aren't.

Eat three meals a day: It took food to put the weight on your body, and it is logical that it will take good food to get it off and to remain healthy while doing so.

Eat only when sitting down: This is something that many Americans find hard to do. Think about those food items that are eaten "on the run." They are usually snack foods such as potato chips, candy bars, and ice cream that are loaded with calories but will leave you hungry in a short while. If you had to go to the table with a plate and a napkin and sit down to eat a bag of potato chips, would you do it? Of course not. So when you eat, you must do it while sitting down at a table.

Weigh yourself every morning and keep a weight chart: Every morning right after you get out of bed, weigh yourself. Record your weight on your weight chart and the requirements for Rule 3 are completed.

It is so exciting to see the pounds go down as you stay on this diet. One important thing to remember is that you should weigh yourself on the same scale each day because sometimes another scale may be off and you will think you have gained or lost weight when you haven't. You could become discouraged and go off the diet just from the results of a scale that is calibrated incorrectly. Don't chance it. Stick to your own scale.

Eat at the same time every day: Rule 4 may be hard for you to follow. Many of us are in the habit of skipping meals, and we also have hectic schedules that make eating at the same time each day difficult. Plan what time of the day you want to eat each of your meals and try your best not to change the times. Be certain not to miss even one meal.

Eat slowly: You should take at least twenty-five minutes to eat each of the meals. I know that sometimes you will feel pressured by a demanding schedule and you will fall back into the old habit of eating quickly, but this is one of the main reasons you are overweight. You need to give your stomach time to tell your brain that it is full. Try not to cheat on this rule.

No caffeine: Did you know that caffeine makes you hungry? You do not need anything that will stimulate your appetite when you are on a diet. So give up all foods that contain caffeine, including coffee, tea, chocolate, and most colas. Be sure to read the label on the aspirin you take. Most tablets contain caffeine, but you can find some that do not. If you are a smoker all I ask is that you cut down the number of cigarettes you smoke each day by half.

Take a multivitamin each day: There is a lot of controversy about vitamins, but one can't hurt you. You may also want to take a vitamin called biotin. It helps the body burn calories. You can purchase it at any health food store.

Drink lots of water: Drink at least 8 glasses of water every day in addition to the other beverages you may drink. It is very important that you keep your body well hydrated.

Don't salt your food: You do not need to add salt to your diet when the foods you eat already contain natural salts. Take the salt shaker off the table. You can use a salt substitute if you like, but I have found them to have such a bitter potassium taste that the food usually tastes better without it. It will take just a few days to get used to using less salt and then your craving for it will disappear.

I'm not asking you to give up salt completely—just cut down on its use. Like fat, all Americans probably eat too much salt. Four to 6 grams, and occasionally 8 to 10 grams of salt a day, will not be harmful to a person in good health. Salt does have important functions, one of which is to retain water in your body. An excess of salt will cause us to retain more than the optimum amount of water, which can lead to a rapid weight gain; this problem is particularly acute for women directly before and during menstruation. It is not within the scope of this book to discuss the role of salt in high blood pressure and other health-related problems. Just remember that if you consume a lot of salt and you drink water, you can expect the body to retain that water for thirty to thirty-six hours. Reduce the intake of salt, and the body will release the water. So . . . don't get waterlogged and cut down on the salt.

These simple rules are the real key to a successful weight-loss program. Combine them with the fifteen-minute exercise program found at the end of the book, and the six weeks will melt away as quickly as your extra pounds.

Questions Most Frequently Asked

Q. Sometimes I get hunger pains and I just can't stand it. Is this normal and will they go away?

A. It is normal for the first two or three days to have hunger pains. They won't last long, however. You have to remember that you were probably eating over 6,000 calories a day and that now you are down to 1,200 to 900 calories a day. It will take just a few days for your stomach to adjust to its daily ration.

Q. Will I get constipated?

A. I found that many of the midshipmen suffered from this problem at the very beginning. They weren't drinking all the water they were supposed to drink. If you keep up your fluid intake the problem will probably diminish. Eating bran cereal in any form (muffins, pancakes) at one meal each day also helps.

Q. Why isn't there any milk on this diet? Should I still drink my glass of milk every day?

A. Humans are the only mammals who continue to drink milk after they are weaned. Calcium is essential to our well-being, but milk is just one source of calcium. The Annapolis Diet includes both milk and cheese in many of the recipes. Fish and potatoes also contain calcium. Because some of the midshipmen were still growing and because of their activity level, we tried to keep the calcium level as high as possible, aiming for an intake of 800 milligrams per day. In any case, the daily requirement of calcium can usually be supplied by the vitamin pill to be taken everyday.

Think of cow's milk like this: When you break it down, you get water, sugar (lactose), and fat. So you're drinking sugar water with butter (fat) in it. Sounds revolting, doesn't it?

Q. I'm a woman and still menstruating. Will I gain weight during menstruation even though I'm sticking to the diet?

A. Many women gain a few pounds just prior to menstruation because of fluid retention. This is normal, and it will happen when you are on the diet. During that time you will probably notice those extra pounds, but don't panic and eat. Just wait a few days and you will be rewarded with a weight loss.

Q. Is the Annapolis Diet low in cholesterol?

A. Yes, the Annapolis Diet is very low in cholesterol. Each recipe has the cholesterol calculated for you. Unfortunately, most of the foods that are high in cholesterol are also high in the protein your body needs. You should consume between 45 and 55 grams of protein per day. Most Americans do so by eating lots of red meat, but meat is high in cholesterol. Yet there are other sources of protein that are low in cholesterol—fish, chicken, and egg whites among them. Stick to these during—and after—your diet. Just remember that shellfish is high in cholesterol and if you are on a low-cholesterol diet you should avoid lobster, crab, and shrimp.

Q. Can I have my evening cocktail and still lose weight?

A. Yes, but please make it a wine spritzer or a light brandy and soda. You could also have a gin with sugarless tonic.

Q. What if I have a chocoholic attack and have to have a candy bar?

A. We aren't perfect all of the time. Cut the candy bar into eight pieces. Eat one piece. Your craving should be satisfied. Now freeze the other pieces for your next attack, but just make sure it's not on the same day! Remember that there are approximately 270 calories in that candy bar and 33½ calories in that one little piece!

Q. What if I get dizzy while I'm on the diet?

A. You may feel a little dizzy the first two days of this diet. This dizziness will go away. It is probably caused by a slight shift in your body fluid. Remember that you'll lose about 7 pounds the first week, and 5 of these pounds are probably water. Getting up fast from a sitting or lying position can cause a momentary drop in blood pressure because you have sustained a slight loss of blood volume due to the water loss. This will sometimes make you woozy. It is not serious and will go away as your body reregulates itself.

If you do get dizzy, eat an orange. An orange is a quick source of potassium, which will alleviate the dizziness. If your dizzy spells continue past the first few days, contact your doctor.

Q. When eating out, is there a basic formula for ordering from the menu?

A. Yes. Order melon first if it's on the menu. Order a salad without dressing and request that they bring you some vinegar. You can have one cracker with the salad. Then order broiled fish or chicken. Don't order anything with a sauce.

Q. I have a hard time staying on the diet on weekends. How can I stick to it without fasting?

A. Just be careful what you put in your mouth. For breakfast stick to the Rush Hour menu. Have salad and a piece of melon for lunch. Then for dinner you can really enjoy yourself. But as we said earlier, make it 4 ounces of broiled fish or chicken, 2 cups of salad greens, and no more than ½ cup of rice. Again, have a slice of cantaloupe for dessert, and you will not have exceeded the calorie count for the day.

Q. Can I lose weight faster by severely cutting back the number of calories provided by the Annapolis Diet?

A. Of course you can, but nine chances out of ten you will cut back for one or two days and then go on a binge to reward yourself. In the end you will gain all of your weight back and then some. You must learn to eat properly and consistently in the correct portions.

Q. What if I stay on the diet, but I just don't lose weight?

A. If you honestly stay on the diet for two weeks and you haven't lost any weight, then you should consult your physician.

Q. Why should I weigh myself every day?

A. You need to weigh yourself every day so that you can see your progress. It is a daily reward. If possible weigh yourself in the morning nude.

Q. Will I see a weight loss every day on the Annapolis Diet?

A. Some days you won't lose that pound you expected to lose. Several midshipmen did not lose for three days and then in one day lost 3 pounds. Sometimes when the weather is hot you may experience some fluid retention and not lose. Just stick with it; if you follow the plan you will lose the weight.

Q. Do I have to give up cigarettes?

A. I am a nonsmoker so my standard answer is, "I hope so." But I realize that you can't always just quit. Just remember that your body can do without all of that nicotine, which is a stimulant. Furthermore, most heavy smokers also drink pots of coffee every day, and the stimulant in coffee—caffeine—is not allowed on this diet. It really makes you hungry.

Q. Why can I have only two diet sodas a day? I usually have six or eight.

A. Diet soda doesn't have any calories, but it is loaded with sodium, so it will be harder to lose weight if you drink lots of soda. So I say, two diet sodas are enough. Drink water instead.

Q. I'm on high blood pressure pills and my doctor told me that this could cause a loss of potassium. Will the melon help replace it?

A. Yes. There are lots of other foods high in potassium, orange juice, bananas, and apricots among them.

Q. If I'm overweight, does that mean that I have more fat cells than my skinny friends?

A. Not necessarily. Some authorities believe that you are born with all the fat cells you have. They just stretch and get bigger as you gain weight. Think of them as balloons. Some of them are filled and some aren't. Watch out for those empty fat cells—they are screaming to be filled!

Q. I hate to exercise. How can I make it less work?

A. If you can, get outside and walk. A half-hour walk is good, but an hour-long walk is better. You will feel better, too. Stretching exercises like touching your toes twenty-five times and stretching your arms over your head will help, too. Move your limbs. Try to squeeze in some exercise time for yourself every day and increase your activity level so that you burn 300 extra calories per day.

Q. Do I really have to drink all that water?

A. Yes. It is important to keep your body well hydrated.

Q. I hate vegetables. What else can I have?

A. I always told the midshipmen that they would learn to love their vegetables. Put them in the salad uncooked if that helps. If the menu calls for brussels sprouts and you hate them cooked, then cut them in half raw, put 1 ounce of diet thousand island dressing on them, toss, and I'll bet you'll love them. Use fresh spinach leaves for the salad instead of lettuce. Eat the carrots raw. But no matter what, eat your vegetables. They are a great source of vitamins, especially vitamin A.

Q. I don't eat breakfast. Can I just skip it and eat more for lunch?

A. No. You must eat breakfast. Skipping meals is just a bad habit that you must break now. Your body has had no nourishment for eight hours while you were sleeping. If you skip breakfast, you will overeat at lunch. To quote an old adage: "You should eat breakfast like a king, lunch like a prince, and dinner like a pauper."

Q. I love junk food. Can I use the fast food menus for lunch and dinner if I want and still lose weight?

A. Yes, but only twice a week. Otherwise you may be tempted to treat yourself to a tripleburger!

Q. I live my life in a rush. Can I still lose weight on this diet?

A. It's time for you to schedule for yourself twenty-five minutes three times a day. Let the remaining hours of your life be rushed.

Q. I love snack foods like potato chips, cheese crackers, and nuts and I hate to give them up. What can I do?

A. Switch to dry air–prepared popcorn that is unsalted but seasoned. There are just a little over 20 calories per cup and it will satisfy that need for something crunchy without the calories.

Q. Can I switch the menus from day to day?

A. Yes, just watch the calorie count.

Q. Does everyone lose 7 pounds the first week?

A. Some people have lost as much as 12 pounds. The weight loss will vary, but you will be satisfied with the results if you stay on the diet.

Q. What is the least fattening fish to eat that still tastes good?

A. Steamed clams have only 33 calories in 4 ounces. Boiled crab, shrimp, or lobster have only about 105 calories per 4 ounces. Beware of trout, which has lots of fat and has 273 calories per every 4 ounces versus 80 calories per every 4 ounces of broiled haddock.

Q. If I go to McDonald's, will I save calories by ordering the fish sandwich?

A. No. There are fewer calories in a hamburger.

Q. Why can't I have the chicken skin? It's the best part.

A. That's where the fat is. On a large chicken breast there are about 150 calories in the skin alone.

Q. Can I have hot chocolate?

A. If it is the low-calorie variety. But remember that there is caffeine in chocolate.

Q. Is herb tea all right to drink?

A. Yes; it contains no calories or caffeine.

Q. I need a snack in the evening? What can I have?

A. Any sliced vegetable, a slice of cantaloupe, or dry air–prepared popcorn.

Q. If I feel full before I've finished all the food on a menu, can I leave it?

A. Yes. There are a lot of overweight people in this world because they were taught from early childhood to "clean their plates."

Q. If I just have to have a jumboburger, can I jog later in the day and burn off those calories?

A. Just remember one thing: That hamburger is going to be about 700 or 800 calories, maybe more; you can burn 600 calories an hour jogging. That's a long time to jog.

Q. Do I need to exercise more?

A. Find a way to add enough extra exercise to your daily routine so that you will burn an additional 300 calories per day.

Q. Is there any food I have to eliminate while on the Annapolis Diet?

A. Yes: oils; animal fats like butter, cream, and whole milk; and shortenings. They are high in calories, and there is good evidence that they contribute to atherosclerosis (especially if it runs in your family), which causes death from strokes and heart attacks. Remember: "Little green apples don't fall far from the tree." The time to protect your body from these hereditary tendencies is now.

Q. Why can't I have club soda?

A. Because it is loaded with salt. That is the reason it tastes so good. Become a label reader and you'll be very surprised at the sodium content in foods. Treat yourself to soda water at parties only.

Q. Why should I take biotin, and what is it?

A. Biotin is a vitamin that is essential to the maintenance of enzyme systems in the body. It helps burn calories. Although the daily minimum requirement has not been established, it is suggested that we consume 150 to 300 micrograms daily. It's found naturally in milk, liver, egg yolks, and yeast. It is also available in tablet form in most drug stores or health food stores.

Q. I really need my coffee in the morning. Can't I just have that?

A. Yes, as long as it is decaffeinated.

Q. Why do I have to eat melon?

A. Because it satisfies the sweet tooth. Also, the fructose, potassium, and high amounts of vitamins A and C it contains make you feel good. It has fewer calories than grapefruit. Its sweetness keeps you coming back for more. A large amount still has few calories—a real plus.

2

Scales and Charts

Thousands of diets have been devised, and each one promises to be the best. They all seem to guarantee rapid weight loss, which anyone who is overweight desires, but not many of them also give you a lifetime plan for keeping off those unwanted pounds because they do not change your eating habits. In six weeks on the Annapolis Diet you will learn to change the bad habits you have developed, replacing favorite old foods with a list of new favorites that won't make you overweight.

Conversation among dieters usually centers around that one little word *calorie:* How many calories in this and how many calories in that? The advantage of this diet is that all the calories are counted for you. Just prepare the recipes and eat the specified portion and you'll see the results fast.

I know that you have heard it before, but the mathematical approach to weight loss cannot be ignored. To lose one pound of fat you have to eat 3,500 fewer calories than you normally would. Sounds like a lot of calories, doesn't it?

I have a friend who went on a diet and counted the calories he did *not* eat by keeping a very good record. He was astounded by the results. For breakfast he normally ate two eggs, two pieces of white toast, four strips of bacon, a large glass of orange juice, and hot chocolate. He reduced his breakfast to one egg, one piece of toast, one strip of low-calorie bacon, and ¼ glass orange juice and substituted herb tea for the hot chocolate. By doing so, he discovered that he had saved himself over 600 calories, and that was just at breakfast. See how those nasty calories add up fast?

He always had a business lunch with friends. He usually started with three martinis and then ordered soup, salad, a steak sandwich, and apple pie for dessert. To reduce his caloric intake, he substituted soda water for the three martinis. He decided to have the soup without the crackers. He used vinegar on his salad and ate the steak sandwich without the bread. He ordered a wedge of melon instead of apple pie for dessert. Just by using good sense, he saved himself 1,135 calories at lunch. If he were to have cut back in the same way at dinner, he would have saved enough calories to have lost 1 pound in just one day. See how it works?

I don't want this chapter to become a health lesson, but there are a few basics you need to understand. Here is a simple way to calculate how many calories it takes to maintain your body weight under normal levels of activity. If you want to weigh 125 pounds, multiply 125 by 15. That equals 1,875. That means that to maintain your weight at 125 pounds, you need 1,875 calories per day. If you are over twenty-five years of age and less active, multiply the desired weight by 11 instead. You will need fewer calories to maintain the same weight as you grow older.

If you normally eat hearty meals and snacks that add up to 3,500 calories per day, cut down your intake to 1,200 calories and you will eventually weight 125 pounds. Go on the 900-calorie diet in this book and you'll lose even faster. The following tables will show you your correct weight, the recommended caloric intake to maintain it, and how many calories various activites burn.

HEIGHT/WEIGHT SCREENING TABLE

HEIGHT Feet	Inches	MEN Range	WOMEN Range
4	10		87-126
4	11		89-128
5	0	100-153	92-130
5	1	102-155	95-132
5	2	103-158	97-134
5	3	104-160	100-136
5	4	105-164	103-139
5	5	106-169	106-144
5	6	109-174	108-148
5	7	111-179	111-152
5	8	115-184	114-156
5	9	119-189	117-161
5	10	123-194	119-165
5	11	127-199	122-169
6	0	131-205	125-174
6	1	135-211	128-179
6	2	139-218	130-185
6	3	143-224	133-190
6	4	147-230	136-196
6	5	151-236	139-201
6	6	153-242	141-206
6	7	157-248	144-211
6	8	166-254	147-216

Our advice at the Naval Academy is that to stay healthy while dieting, you should not allow your caloric intake to fall short of 900 calories. Most physicians suggest that you should stay on a diet lower than 800 calories per day for absolutely no longer than two weeks. Remember—you are trying to lose fat. A drastically reduced diet will cause you to lose muscle as well. Always consult your physician before starting any diet.

RECOMMENDED CALORIC INTAKE TO MAINTAIN WEIGHT _____

HEIGHT		AVERAGE WEIGHT		MODERATE ACTIVITY	VERY ACTIVE
Feet	Inches	Men	Women	Men/Women	Men/Women
5	2	123	113	1353/1243	1845/1695
5	3	127	116	1397/1276	1905/1740
5	4	130	120	1430/1320	1950/1800
5	5	133	123	1463/1353	1995/1845
5	6	136	128	1496/1408	2040/1920
5	7	140	132	1540/1452	2100/1980
5	8	145	136	1595/1496	2175/2040
5	9	149	140	1639/1540	2235/2100
5	10	153	144	1683/1584	2295/2160
5	11	158	148	1738/1628	2370/2220
6	0	162	152	1782/1672	2430/2280
6	1	166		1826	2490
6	2	171		1881	2565
6	3	176		1936	2640

I had 30 extra pounds "sneak" up on me. Oh, it was 5 pounds here and 5 pounds there. My size 12 dresses were getting snug, so I just bought a few size 14s and that became my new dress size. I gradually accepted those few extra pounds until I weighed 30 pounds more than what I had always weighed since I was twenty-five. I knew I had to get serious about dieting or I would arrive at 200 pounds fast. It really scared me. So I started keeping track of my calories. I hated grapefruit, sliced tomatoes, and bland food in general, so I decided I would spice up my diet food. I used half a bottle of red pepper flakes in two weeks, but my mouth was happy. I was cooking and eating all day and I was losing weight.

CALORIES BURNED FOR 30 MINUTES OF EXERCISE _____

ACTIVITY	CALORIES 150-pound person	CALORIES 125-pound person
Walking	105	90
Jogging	324	250
Bicycling	150	120
Dancing	126	100
Basketball	210	180
Football	291	250
Golf	90	70
Bedmaking	142	140
Office work	60	46
Watching TV	53	40
Skating	250	200
Skiing	390	325
Swimming	307	240
Tennis	250	200
General housework	123	90
Standing at attention	60	40
Sleeping	36	20

What a fantastic combination for this "blimpy" gourmet! I cooked the same food for my family and just gave them larger portions. So they never really noticed I was dieting.

It's easy to stick to this diet. Still, it's essential to know how many calories are in foods other than those on this controlled diet. Often you'll have to eat out or with friends.

Here are several lists for handy reference. The charts will help keep you on course over the next six weeks. If you cheat on the diet check with the chart to see how much it will cost you in terms of calories. Then all you have to do the next day is to go back on the diet. You don't have to confess to anyone that you cheated—you know it!

A QUICK REFERENCE TO THE CALORIC CONTENT
OF COMMON FOODS _____

Item	Amount	Calories
BEVERAGES		
Hot chocolate	6 ounces	206
Cola	10 ounces	129
Diet soda	16 ounces	1
Ginger ale	10 ounces	106
Milk	8 ounces	152
ALCOHOLIC BEVERAGES		
Beer	12 ounces	155
Red wine	4 ounces	96
White wine	4 ounces	88
Champagne	4 ounces	100
Gin, 80 proof	1 ounce	65
Bourbon	1 ounce	83
Scotch	1 ounce	70
GRAINS		
Cornflakes	1 cup	112
Puffed rice	1 cup	55
Rice krispies	1 cup	110
All bran	1 cup	120
Rice, cooked	2/3 cup	129
Spaghetti noodles	1 cup	155
Pancake	4-inch	62
Waffle	7-inch	209
French toast	1 slice	85
English muffin	1	130
Bagel	1	165
White bread	1 slice	63
Whole rye bread	1 slice	75
Diet rye bread	1 slice	30
Corn grits	1/2 cup	122

Item	Amount	Calories
MEAT, POULTRY, AND SEAFOODS		
Ground sirloin, broiled	4 ounces	248
Lamb chop, broiled	5 ounces	122
Porterhouse steak, before cooking	16 ounces	372
Rump roast	4 ounces	236
Sirloin steak, lean	4 ounces	268
Chuck pot roast	4 ounces	243
Veal cutlet	4 ounces	245
Chicken breast, before cooking	8 ounces	197
Roasting chicken	4 ounces	206
Duck, meat only	4 ounces	187
Turkey	4 ounces	200
Blue fish, broiled	4 ounces	199
Clams	4 ounces	33
Cod	4 ounces	193
Crab, steamed	4 ounces	105
Flounder, baked	4 ounces	229
Haddock, broiled	4 ounces	80
Lobster, meat only	4 ounces	108
Oysters	4 ounces	86
Salmon	4 ounces	119
Shrimp	4 ounces	103
Sole	4 ounces	90
Tuna	4 ounces	120
Trout	4 ounces	273
VEGETABLES		
Asparagus	1/2 cup	20
Bean sprouts	1/2 cup	19
Beets	1/2 cup	30
Broccoli	1/2 cup	77
Brussels sprouts	4 ounces	37
Cabbage	1/2 cup	11
Carrots	1/2 cup	24
Cauliflower	1/2 cup	14
Celery	1/2 cup	10
Cucumber	1/2 cup	10

Item	Amount	Calories
Eggplant	½ cup	19
Green beans	½ cup	13
Mushrooms	½ cup	10
Onions, sliced	½ cup	21
Peas	½ cup	57
Peppers, green	½ cup	16
Potato, baked	1 small	92
Spinach	½ cup	26
Squash	½ cup	19
Tomato	1 small	24
Zucchini	½ cup	9

FRUITS

Apple	1 medium	66
Apricots, whole	3	55
Avocado	1	302
Banana	1	81
Blueberries	½ cup	45
Cantaloupe, medium	½ melon	82
Cantaloupe	½ cup	24
Grapes, fresh	½ cup	52
Grapefruit	½	74
Orange	1	77
Peach	1	38
Pear	1	101
Pineapple	2 slices	66
Plum	1	27
Rhubarb	½ cup	10
Strawberries	1 cup	53
Watermelon	1 cup	42

FRUIT JUICES

Grapefruit juice	½ cup	48
Orange juice	½ cup	56
Pineapple juice, sweetened	½ cup	64
Tomato juice	½ cup	23

Item	Amount	Calories
Apple juice	1/2 cup	61
Apple cider	1/2 cup	58
Vegetable juice cocktail	1/2 cup	19

CONDIMENTS

Mustard	3 teaspoons	3
Ketchup	1 tablespoon	24
Jam/jelly	1 tablespoon	54
Sugar	1 tablespoon	46
Mayonnaise	1 tablespoon	101
All oils	1 tablespoon	124
Peanut butter	1 tablespoon	100
A-1 sauce	1 tablespoon	13
Cocktail sauce	1 tablespoon	24
Sour cream	1 tablespoon	26
Soy sauce	1 tablespoon	6
Taco sauce	1 tablespoon	4
Tarter sauce	1 tablespoon	75
Worcestershire sauce	1 tablespoon	10
Butter	1 tablespoon	102

DAIRY PRODUCTS

Yogurt, low fat, flavored	1 cup	270
Ice milk	1/2 cup	99
Sherbet	1/4 pint	130
Half and half	1 tablespoon	22
Egg, large	1	77
Cheddar cheese	1 ounce	83
American cheese	1 ounce	70
Swiss cheese	1 ounce	97
Cottage cheese, 2 percent	1/2 cup	77

SNACK FOOD CALORIE COUNTER

Frankfurter	1	136
Saltine cracker	8	88
"Ritz" cracker	1	17

Item	Amount	Calories
Chocolate chip cookie	1	80
Popcorn, plain	1 cup	23
Potato chips	10	90
Pretzels, medium	1 pretzel	7
Hershey bar	1 small	150
Biscuit	1	103
French fries	10	125

FAST FOOD CALORIE CHART

ARTHUR TREACHER'S FISH & CHIPS

Fish	2 pieces	355
Chips	1 serving	276

BASKIN-ROBBINS

Ice cream	1 scoop	133–148

BURGER KING

Hamburger with cheese	1	347
Whopper with cheese	1	740
Onion rings, large	1 order	331
French fries	1 order, regular	209
Vanilla shake	1	336

DUNKIN DONUTS

Cake donut	1	240
Yeast raised	1	160

HARDEE'S

Ham biscuit	1 order	340
Sausage biscuit	1 order	413
Ham biscuit with egg	1 order	458

JACK IN THE BOX

Hamburger, deluxe	1	260
Jumbo Jack, with cheese	1	628
Regular taco	1	189
Moby Jack sandwich	1	455
Onion rings	1 order	351

Item	Amount	Calories
KENTUCKY FRIED CHICKEN		
Drumstick, original recipe	1 piece	117
Drumstick, extra crispy	1 piece	155
Dinner with drumstick and thigh, roll, mashed potatoes, gravy, cole slaw	Original	643
	Extra crispy	765
LONG JOHN SILVER'S SEAFOOD SHOPPES		
Fish & chips with slaw	3 pieces	1,190
Shrimp with batter	6 pieces	269
Breaded oysters	6 pieces	460
S.O.S. super ocean sandwich	1	554
Corn on the cob	1	174
Hush puppies	3 per order	153
Pecan pie	3 ounces	367
McDONALD'S		
Egg McMuffin	1	352
Hash brown potatoes	1 order	130
Hamburger	1	257
Quarter Pounder with cheese	1	518
Big Mac	1	541
Fillet-o-Fish	1	402
Chocolate shake	1	323
Regular french fries	1 order	209
ORANGE JULIUS		
Orange Julius	12 ounces	149
PIZZA HUT		
Thin 'n' Crispy, 2 pieces, standard	Super cheese	410
	Pepperoni	370
	Super supreme	520
Thick 'n' Chewy, 2 pieces, standard	Super cheese	450
	Pepperoni	450
	Super supreme	590

Item	Amount	Calories
RUSTLER STEAK HOUSE		
(Platters with potato, margarine, roll)		
Rustler strip steak	(Steak only, 337 calories)	878
T-bone steak	(T-bone only, 374 calories)	952
Steak and crab	(Steak & crab only, 479 calories)	1,052
Beef patty	8 ounces	1,001
Clam	1 order	945
Seafood combination	1 order	1,167
Rib eye steak	(Steak only, 224 calories)	802
Salad bar items:		
Lettuce	2 ounces	7
Onions	1 ounce	11
Tomato	2 ounces	13
Cucumbers	½ ounce	2
Radishes	¾ ounce	4
Celery	½ ounce	2
Carrots	¼ ounce	3
Kidney beans	1 ounce	26
Chick peas	1 ounce	102
Green beans	1 ounce	7
Bean sprouts	1 ounce	8
Bac-o-bits	¼ ounce	29
Grated cheese	¼ ounce	29
Green peppers	¾ ounce	5
Dressings:		
Italian, French, Russian	1 tablespoon	60
Blue cheese	1 tablespoon	80
TACO BELL		
Regular taco	1	159
Tostada	1	206

Item	Amount	Calories
Bean burrito	1	345
Enchirito	1	391
Beefy tostada	1	291
Bellbeefer	1	243
Pintos 'n' cheese	1	231

WENDY'S

Hamburger	1 single	472
	1 double	669
	1 single with cheese	577
	1 triple with cheese	1,036
Chili	1 order	229
Frosty	1	391

WHITE CASTLE

Hamburger	1	160
Double cheeseburger	1	305
Fish sandwich, without tartar sauce	1	192
Fish sandwich with cheese	1	217

WIENERSCHNITZEL

Super deluxe	1	472
Corn dog	1	520
Kraut dog	1	241
Chili dog	1	269
Chili cheese dog	1	311

CALORIES IN COMMON RESTAURANT FOOD (approximate)

Plain egg omelet	3 eggs	350
Eggs benedict	1 order	700
Bacon	4 slices	292
Sausage links	4	312
Toast, buttered	2 slices	225
Danish pastry	medium	325

Item	Amount	Calories
Spaghetti with meat sauce	1 order	600
New York strip steak	10 ounces	629
Prime rib au jus	large	730
Lobster, broiled, drawn butter	1¼ pounds	500
Caesar salad	1½ cups	364
Chili	bowl	600
Ice cream	1 scoop	100

3

Diet Plan Menus
for Six Weeks

Now that I have given you all the charts in Chapter 2, you have an easy guide to keep you from going too far astray. Still, you may be asking yourself, "Is it worth it?" Yes, it is. So don't you fool yourself into thinking fat—think thin!

Let's get started. We will begin with your kitchen. Go to the pantry and hide the beans, shortening, and sugar. If you have any boxed cake, cookie, or muffin mixes, turn those boxes around so that you won't see the beautiful picture of the chocolate layer cake or the chocolate chip cookies every time you look in the food pantry. If necessary, put them on the top shelf so that you can't even see the top of the box. Now go to the freezer. Put the ice cream, sweet rolls, and TV dinners on the bottom shelf. Fill large baggies with ice cubes and cover those tempting items with ice. You can use the ice—but not the fattening food under it. If you have an ice maker in the freezer you will have no reason to use the bottom shelf at all. Put the breaded fish on the next shelf up and cover them with frozen fish fillets. On the next shelf up put the frozen vegetables and finally the frozen fruits. Are you getting the picture? Yes, it's a game, but it must be played seriously, for you and your good looks are at stake.

Now let's go to the spice cabinet. If the ground spices are over a year old, discard them. Make a list of these herbs and spices: thyme, basil, tarragon, cloves, oregano, and rosemary. You can add more later, but that's a good start. Be sure that you have garlic powder and onion powder, and a jar of dried parsley will also come in handy. Put the garlic salt, seasoned salt, and meat marinade way in the back, out of reach and out of view. Now put a large can of vegetable spray on the back of the stove, and put the solid vegetable shortening and the cooking oil in the back of the broom closet behind the three-year supply of vacuum cleaner bags. I'm not kidding! You have to make it hard on yourself because we all know that in the beginning the temptation to go back to old habits is incredible. You may feel that you are completely rearranging your kitchen, but if you follow these steps, going back to the old ways is going to take a lot of effort that, hopefully, you won't want to make.

Now let's tackle the refrigerator. Put the mayonnaise, peanut butter, honey, jelly, olives, and mustard in the bottom drawer, which is usually labeled "Fruits." Tell the family that the drawer belongs to them and that they must keep their food there, out of your sight. In full view on the top shelf put the diet salad dressing. Put two bottles of diet soda and two bottles of mineral water next to the salad dressing. And from now on purchase only diet drinks. The children will complain at first, but they will get used to it. Besides, it's better for their teeth. Don't give in! Purchase three heads of lettuce, clean them, and put them in a large plastic bag so that they take up nearly all of the second shelf. Fill a basket with tomatoes, green onions, carrots, and celery that have been cleaned and placed in plastic bags, and put the basket next to the lettuce so that you will always have something to "grab" for. If you feel a binge coming on, at least the lowest calorie food is ready and waiting for you.

Now boil two eggs and chop one dill pickle. Put a large can of tuna fish into a glass dish, chop the hard-cooked eggs, and stir the eggs and pickle into the tuna. Cover tightly and put on the third shelf. You can have ¼ cup of this mixture at a time when the diet just isn't enough. In the meantime, tell the children that all they have to do is add mayonnaise to make their own sandwiches. This mixture will last three days, I predict.

Finally, check the refrigerator carefully for anything else that is forbidden and turn it around, give it to a neighbor, or hide it. But for heaven's sake don't eat it! You are just putting those things away temporarily. It is not forever, just a few weeks. Later you can eat them again in moderation. All skinny people eat ice cream and peanut butter—now and then! Do you get the point? Good.

It's now 10:00 A.M. You have finished rearranging the kitchen and the phone rings. "Sally, this is Martha. Look, I'm just dying to get out of the house today. Let's go to that new little restaurant on Main Street. We can diet tomorrow." Oh, no! Now you have an option. You can lie and tell her you're having four teeth pulled in an hour. Better yet, invite her to your house for lunch to try this new recipe you're making. You can go to that new restaurant soon. I realize that you can't turn your kitchen into the local eatery, but in the beginning it is just less tempting to stay close to home.

Eventually, however, you are going to have to accept those invitations to lunch or dinner. When you are invited, tell the hostess that you are dieting and that it is really working for you. Keep the conversation positive so that she will help you stay on your diet. Remember, on the Annapolis Diet you can eat almost anything. It's the *portion* you have to watch. Let your hostess know that the only things you can't have are fried food and salt. That, of course, is a little oversimplified, but it gives her a world of choices. Tell her not to worry about your salad dressing; you'll just tuck one of your handy diet dressing packets into your purse and give it to her when you arrive. Then no one will know that your salad is special. After all, what are friends for? Share one of your new quick and easy fruit dessert recipes with her and she'll probably serve that for dessert.

You arrive at the party and find that there are fifteen courses, not fried but all bathed in rich creamy sauces—just the ones you love. Take four bites of everything. Discreetly move the sauce from the bites you are going to eat. You'll still be adding calories to your daily intake, but it's not polite to carry on. Then rave and rave about the absolutely fantastic food. Tell the hostess that it's the best dish you've ever had. If she asks why you aren't eating very much, just say that your stomach must have shrunk because of your new diet. She will love you for your compliments and really won't care that you didn't clean your plate. Now, I know that you'll *want* to clean every lick off that plate, but just hold onto your empty fork. Let the hostess clean it off for you—in the kitchen. For dessert, fruit will probably be served, along with the cheese and crackers. Remember, you can have only the fruit!

I know that going out is the most tempting and difficult thing to do while dieting, but you can't become a recluse because you are on a diet. Go out and have fun. In a restaurant, order broiled chicken or fish and salad with vinegar only, or whisk out one of your packets of diet dressing. Order a baked potato. When it arrives, scoop out all the potato and eat only the skin. There are only about 30 calories in the skin and you can well afford them. A refreshing beverage is ice water with a squeeze of fresh lemon in a fancy glass. It really is simple; just stick by these rules and you will still lose. But remember, when they bring you a 12-ounce chicken breast, at least half of that chicken must go home with you in a doggy bag for tomorrow's luncheon salad.

The hardest place to control yourself is at a party or at a restaurant with friends. If you feel you have to order an alcoholic beverage, then order a white wine spritzer. Ask the bartender to make the spritzer with 1 ounce of wine and fill it up with a diet lemon-lime drink or Perrier. That way your drink is only 25 calories instead of 250. Now's the time to order soda water or your favorite diet soda with a slice of lime. You will find that the other guests will never ask you why you are not drinking.

The menus for the fast food restaurants can be substituted for any menu in the book when it becomes necessary to go out for a meal. It is essential that you become familiar with the caloric content of most restaurant foods so that you are never caught off guard and upon arriving home find that you have just eaten for dinner all the calories allowed for the entire day!

Glance through the menus and you will find that the foods included here are really tasty. You won't be suffering too much. I have tried to include your favorite foods, but I have left out all the fried foods. My guess is that you will learn to love these foods and that you will therefore stay thin forever.

The menus in this book were designed to give you as much variety as possible. I don't expect you to change your entire life-style just because you have a few pounds to lose. Thus, the recipes presented here use those ingredients that have the fewest calories but afford the finest flavor. The menus will serve as a guide. You can easily see the caloric count for each recipe. Make substitutions when desired, but substitute a vegetable recipe for another vegetable or a fish for a fish. This will add variety without changing the caloric or vitamin intake.

Each day you can drink all the low-calorie broth you wish. Look for the calorie count on the box. It should be 18 calories or less per cup. You can also have two cups of lettuce anytime you like. If the hunger pains are getting to you, or you have just got to have something to eat, then head for the refrigerator and have a salad. If you are out for lunch you can usually find an inexpensive salad bar at nearly every fast food restaurant. Eat only the lettuce or the spinach leaves and be sure to use only vinegar or your packets of diet dressing.

Most people need an occasional snack when they begin to diet. I suggest snacking on sliced green peppers, carrots, celery, or sliced cucumber. These won't add too many calories. If you are desperate for chocolate, remember my hint about buying one candy bar, dividing it into eight pieces, wrapping each section individually, and freezing them. When one of those desperate cravings comes along, reach in and take out one piece. It usually helps satisfy the need. See how many days you can go without eating a piece of your precious ration. Save one piece as a treat for yourself on the day you reach your goal.

As I have mentioned, dry air–prepared popcorn makes a nice snack without adding too many calories. Don't add salt but sprinkle it with a little dehydrated American cheese or grated Parmesan cheese. You can also sprinkle it with chili powder, onion powder, or garlic powder. These will add a fraction of the calories that butter will. If you simply must "butter" the popcorn, use only diet margarine and be sure to add the calories into the day's calorie count. Now that is a good deal! When dieting, you must look at every little thing from the positive side.

If you are used to an evening cocktail, have it. But make it with ½ ounce of liquor or 1 ounce of wine and diet soda, soda water, or water. Then use only vinegar on your salad and take half as much of the entree as you normally would. Everything is a trade-off. Of course, sometimes it is relaxing to put up your feet and enjoy a beer or a glass of wine. I'm all for it. If you are of age you can have that special item now and then. Just add the calories to your caloric intake for that day and stay within your desired range. But remember one thing: It is fattening to get drunk. One glass of wine is enough for anyone, especially if you are on a diet.

Almost every recipe in this book can be frozen. Cook a week's worth of dinners on the weekend. Wrap the food carefully and freeze. Now the burden of dieting is even smaller, for you are not in the kitchen as much the other six days of the week. Furthermore, you will begin to learn a lifetime pattern of living with good food.

As you can see, there is a lot of leeway in this diet. So even when dieting you can cope with the demands of everyday life.

The midshipmen found that the most difficult time for dieting was in the evening. They were kept so busy during the day that the opportunity for snacking was very slight. The evening hours, however, allowed time for cheating. You, too, will find that you've developed the habit of eating at one particular time of day when it is not necessary. To solve this problem, I asked the midshipmen to keep a diary of everything they ate every day of the diet, passing out forms for them to use. Eating patterns thus emerged. To determine your own eating pattern, you should also keep a diary the first week of the diet. Put down everything you eat and then read it carefully to see your weak point during the day. To solve the problem, schedule a twenty-minute walk at that time every day. Walk at a brisk pace, and when you return home or to your job, your hunger pains will have vanished. Start today and see if I am right.

Stick to the diet and you will lose weight. As I've said, expect about a 7-pound loss the first week and a 5-pound loss the second. Don't kid yourself into believing that it's all fat. It's not. Much of it is water. You have stopped adding salt to your food, which makes a difference. The third week you may lose only 2 pounds, but you will continue to lose. The midshipmen had plateaus along the way, going several days without shedding a pound. They were tempted to stop eating for several days, but that really doesn't help. To keep your weight down, you must learn how to eat correctly. During plateaus, don't become discouraged or depressed. It will help to increase your out-of-doors activity. Go for a walk or jog. Get outside and move around!

If you are a woman, don't despair if you see a slight

weight gain around the time you are due to menstruate. Just wait a couple of days. It is caused by water retention and will go away. You'll be just fine.

If you are a man and you've combined "pumping iron" (working out with weights) with the diet, you may see the weight come off a bit more slowly. That doesn't mean that you are not losing fat, only building heavy muscles. Muscle weighs more than fat. Just stick to the diet and keep working out.

Two sets of menus are presented here. The first set will provide you with approximately 900 calories per day; the second set consists of maintenance menus providing 1,200 calories per day. These maintenance menus, which are more elaborate, can be scaled down to provide 900 calories a day. Just omit the items that are in italics. Eat all of the other items for each meal. The number in parentheses is the total caloric count for the 900-calorie diet for that meal. The number not in parentheses is the total if you've chosen the 1,200-calorie plan.

The menu is waiting for you. I promise you won't ever go hungry.

Weeks 1 and 2

APPROXIMATELY 900 CALORIES

The Rush Hour Breakfast and Commuter's Lunch menus were added to this diet to make it convenient for the working person. We did not use these at the Naval Academy. These recipes were used by the midshipmen on weekends when they were away from the academy. If you do not work in an office, you can go to the Maintenance Menus and choose the 900-calorie menu for breakfast and lunch if you want to and have the time to do the extra cooking.

The first week is the hardest. But you will love the Raspberry Soup, and the fish entrée for dinner goes together so fast you won't believe it. That's why I put it on the menu three nights a week. You may hate fish, but you will love this recipe. Remember to eat the melon specified in each menu; the high potassium and vitamins will make you feel good. The menus afford a great variety in vegetables, meat, fish, and poultry; the melon is just the "frosting on the cake," so to speak. The third and fourth weeks will offer even more variety.

Monday, Wednesday, Friday

RUSH HOUR BREAKFAST

¼ cantaloupe	24	
⅓ cup granola (no milk)	130	
4 ounces fruit juice	58	212

COMMUTER'S LUNCHEON

1 cup chicken broth	10	
Deli Reuben sandwich	325	
¼ cantaloupe	24	359

DINNER

Raspberry Melon Soup	64	
Lettuce Hearts	17	
2 ounces diet dressing	32	
Cod Cohasset	193	
Potato Skins	33	
Watermelon slice	42	381

DAILY TOTAL: 952 calories

Tuesday, Saturday

BREAKFAST

Orange Melon Juice	85	
Soft-boiled Egg	73	
1 slice whole wheat toast	40	198

LUNCH

1 cup watermelon	42	
Chef's Salad	124	
5 diet melba rounds	50	
Karen's Oranges	128	344

DINNER

Consommé with Melon	18	
Baked Herbed Chicken	173	
Carrots Vichy	12	
Baked potato	92	
Garlic Sticks	56	
Sliced casaba melon	24	375

DAILY TOTAL: 917 calories

Thursday, Sunday

BREAKFAST

¼ cantaloupe	24	
Diet Pancakes	140	
Diet syrup	16	
1 ounce Canadian-style bacon	40	220

LUNCH

1 cup onion broth	10	
Tostada Salad	180	
1 slice honeydew melon	24	214

DINNER

Chicken broth	10	
Beef Shish Kabob	261	
Tossed Romaine Salad	35	
Rice Pilaf	124	
¼ cantaloupe	24	454

DAILY TOTAL: 888 calories

Weeks 3 and 4

You've made it through weeks one and two! I'll bet you are down 12 to 15 pounds. Don't you feel proud of yourself? What a difference a pound makes.

Now let's add some more great dishes this week. You'll have lamb chops three times a week now. The Red Snapper with Melon is just delicious. Invite a friend to share this menu with you. The breakfast menus are repeated, so they should be easy to prepare.

Your weight loss will now slow down a little. Don't expect to lose more than 2 or 3 pounds a week. Don't be discouraged if this is all you lose. This is all you are *expected* to lose. Losing weight gradually is the only healthy way to diet. It is also a good way to fool your body into thinking that it likes your eating this way. If you take it off slowly you probably won't gain it back. So don't be tempted to cut back on your caloric intake. Just enjoy yourself every morning when you weigh yourself.

Monday, Wednesday, Friday

BREAKFAST

Repeat Weeks 1 & 2		212

LUNCH

1 cup beef broth	10	
Bacon, lettuce, tomato sandwich	273	
Dill pickle	15	
1 slice watermelon	42	340

DINNER

1 cup onion broth	10	
Lettuce Hearts	17	
2 ounces diet dressing	24	
1 Broiled Lamb Chop	140	
½ cup Steamed Rice	79	
Baked Tomatoes Parmesan	52	
1 slice melon	24	338

DAILY TOTAL: **890 calories**

Tuesday, Saturday

BREAKFAST

Repeat Weeks 1 & 2		198

LUNCH

1 cup vegetable broth	10	
Chicken sandwich	210	
Sliced casaba melon	24	244

DINNER

1 cup chicken broth	10	
Spinach Melon Salad	59	
Baked Red Snapper with Melon	221	
Potatoes au Gratin	76	
Fresh zucchini	9	
Chive Biscuits	65	
½ cup sliced strawberries	27	481

DAILY TOTAL: 923 calories

Thursday, Sunday

BREAKFAST

Repeat Weeks 1 & 2		220

LUNCH

¼ cantaloupe	24	
1 cup onion broth	10	
Chef's Salad	124	158

DINNER

1 cup beef broth	10	
Italian Salad	65	
Veal Marsala	217	
½ cup pasta	115	
Crookneck Squash	8	
Garlic Bread	66	
Watermelon slice	42	523

DAILY TOTAL: 901 calories

Weeks 5 and 6

Wow! I'll bet you're down about 19 pounds. Aren't you excited to start a new menu this week? I've put Gibson's Loaf on the menu for three days at lunch. You can make one loaf and slice it as the week goes by. It's really tasty and always ready just for you.

As with weeks three and four, you'll lose about 2 pounds a week, but that is all you should lose. The weeks have gone by fast, haven't they? There was nothing to it. I'm really proud of you, and you should be proud of yourself. Now just stick to it and you'll be ready to start the Maintenance Menus in two weeks. You will then be able to eat about 1,200 calories and still lose a little more as you go. Remember, this is a healthful diet that you can follow forever. It's actually a shame to call it a diet.

Monday, Wednesday, Friday

RUSH HOUR BREAKFAST

4 ounces fruit juice	58	
1 slice melon	24	
1 piece thin rye toast	40	
⅓ cup granola	130	252

COMMUTER'S LUNCH

1 cup onion broth	10	
Gibson's Loaf on thin rye	253	
½ cup melon balls	24	287

DINNER

1 cup onion broth	10	
Cabbage Melon Salad	42	
Baked Herbed Chicken	173	
Parmesan Potato Wedges	105	
Chocolate Mousse	54	384

DAILY TOTAL: 923 calories

Tuesday, Saturday

BREAKFAST

¼ cantaloupe	24	
Piperade	94	118

LUNCH

1 slice melon	24	
Tuna salad sandwich	292	
Lettuce Hearts	17	
2 ounces diet dressing	24	357

DINNER

1 cup chicken broth	10	
Red-Leaf Lettuce Salad	28	
3 ounces London Broil	232	
½ cup Rice Pilaf	124	
½ cup carrot nuggets	24	
¼ cantaloupe	24	430

DAILY TOTAL: **905 calories**

Thursday, Sunday

BREAKFAST

Broiled Grapefruit with Melon	68	
Cheese Omelet	131	
1 slice toast	40	
1 slice Canadian-style bacon	40	265

LUNCH

1 cup beef broth	10	
Swiss cheese sandwich	260	
¼ cantaloupe and ⅓ cup strawberries	41	311

DINNER

1 cup vegetable broth	10	
Lettuce Hearts	17	
1 ounce diet dressing	12	
Shrimp Scampi	224	
Sliced tomatoes	35	
½ cup cantaloupe	24	322

DAILY TOTAL: 898 calories

Gourmet Maintenance Diet Menus

At last you've made it. Your new skinny self deserves a little more of this good food. Some of these menus require more cooking, but if you don't want to go to so much trouble, pick out something to substitute from the menus provided for the first six weeks. Now that you know what to do, you don't need me anymore. Just remember that it is not necessarily what you eat that makes you gain weight, it is how much of it you put in your mouth. If you gain a little, go back to the menus for week one and two immediately. Enjoy yourself, and happy eating!

Week 1

Monday, Wednesday, Friday

1,147 CALORIES (946)

BREAKFAST   252 calories (194)
Melon Slush
Fried Egg
2 slices diet toast
1 slice Canadian bacon

LUNCH   318 calories (246)
Chicken Soup
Lettuce Hearts
Diet dressing
Linguini and Melon in Clam Sauce
Carrots Vichy
Garlic Sticks
Apple Sweet

DINNER   577 calories (506)
Seafood Cocktail
Tossed Romaine Salad
Leg of Lamb
Potato Skins
1/2 cup fresh broccoli
Chive Biscuits
Honeydew Whip

Tuesday, Thursday, Sunday

1,204 CALORIES (891)

BREAKFAST   255 calories (255)
Melon Freeze
Cheese Omelet
1 slice rye toast

LUNCH   492 calories (255)
Onion broth
Cabbage Melon Salad
Salisbury Steak and Mushrooms
   or Shrimp Louis
Potatoes au Gratin
Braised Celery
Chocolate Mousse

DINNER   457 calories (381)
Chicken broth
Bean sprout salad
Melon Brown Rice Pilaf
Baked Fillet of Sole
Zucchini and Tomatoes
Sliced melon

Saturday

1,164 CALORIES (886)

BREAKFAST   310 calories (190)
Apple Melon Bake
   or ¼ cantaloupe
3 Diet Pancakes
1 ounce diet syrup

LUNCH   275 calories (275)
Melon Grape Freeze
Tostada Salad
Blueberry Melon Fluff

DINNER   609 calories (421)
Cantaloupe Soup
Beef Shish Kabob
Rice Pilaf
Garlic Bread
Baked eggplant
Strawberry Mousse

Week 2

Monday, Wednesday, Friday

1,144 CALORIES (929)

BREAKFAST   230 calories (230)
Melon Shake
French Toast
Diet syrup

LUNCH   410 calories (348)
German Salad
Leg of Lamb
1/2 cup zucchini
Saffron Rice
Garlic Bread
Raspberry Melon Parfait

DINNER   504 calories (351)
Vegetable Soup
Baked Herbed Chicken
Red Cabbage
Baked potato
Chive Biscuits
Watermelon Mousse

Tuesday, Thursday, Sunday

1,113 CALORIES (925)

BREAKFAST   247 calories (154)
Melon Cup
Poached egg
1 slice Canadian bacon
English muffin
   or ½ English muffin

LUNCH   305 calories (305)
Greek Salad
Broiled Lamb Chop
Risotto
Sautéed Cucumbers
1 slice casaba melon

DINNER   561 calories (466)
Chicken Gumbo Soup
Crab Imperial
Shells with Peas and Mushrooms
Belgian Endive
¼ melon

Saturday

1,241 CALORIES (881)

BREAKFAST   256 calories (156)
Tangerine Melon Boat
Mexican Puff
Flour tortilla

LUNCH   486 calories (305)
Maryland Crab Soup
Spinach Melon Salad
Broiled Red Snapper with Melon
Crookneck Squash
Orange Soufflé

DINNER   499 calories (420)
Karen's Oranges in Melon Cup
Endive Salad
Lamb Shish Kabob
Steamed Rice
Lemon Custard

4

Commuter's and Brown Bagger's Menus

For the working person, sticking to a special diet is almost impossible at lunchtime. American luncheon favorites such as huge deli sandwiches, hamburgers, and steak sandwiches are loaded with calories, while the famous brown bag lunch becomes boring. As always, the challenge is to satisfy the taste buds and the hunger pains while keeping the caloric intake at 350 calories or less. I know how tough it can be.

I've heard many working people say, "I can't stay on a diet because I have to work." It is hard, but here are a few hints that should help.

If you have thirty minutes to an hour for lunch, spend the first half of your lunch break walking. Go anywhere; just get completely out of your working area and walk at a good, fast pace. You will be amazed to discover your hunger level going down markedly. Use the remaining time to eat your lunch slowly.

You can go to the local deli or restaurant and still follow the diet. If you are careful in your ordering, you won't wreck the entire diet by dining out.

Use this chapter as a guide for preparing your lunch. Choose one of the commuter's/brown bagger's menus or a restaurant menu. Do not cheat. If temptation wins, keep track of those extra luncheon calories and deduct them from your dinner menu. Managing your calories is just like managing your money. If you overspend in one area, you must make it up somewhere else. Just don't allow your work to become your excuse for being fat. It is possible to eat at work and lose weight.

Commuter's/Brown Bagger's Menus

Week 1

Monday
Gibson's Loaf Sandwich
Cucumber Salad
Fresh fruit

Tuesday
Chicken Pâté
Sliced Swiss cheese
French bread stick
Melon slices

Wednesday
Cobb Salad Sandwich
Cauliflower vinaigrette
Sliced strawberries

Thursday
Watercress Sandwich
Artichoke Salad
1 slice melon

Friday
1 cup tomato soup
Danish Sea Sandwich
1 apple

Week 2

Monday
Radish salad
Watercress Sandwich with Swiss
    Cheese
1 slice melon

Tuesday
1 cup chicken broth
Duck Salad
Melon and ham

Wednesday
Veal and Ham Terrine
Marinated broccoli
Pineapple and oranges

Thursday
Shrimp and Scallop Salad
Garlic Sticks
1 slice honeydew melon

Friday
Seviche Acapulco
1 wedge Quiche Lorraine
1 slice cantaloupe

Deli Food Menus

In making the calculations in this section, I assumed that you order a regular sandwich with white or rye bread, tomato slices, and lettuce. You can add sliced onion and 1 teaspoon mustard. You should, however, ask that no mayonnaise be put on the sandwich. You can then add your own diet mayonnaise, which you should bring from home. Most delis put five to six ounces or more of meat on their sandwiches. Be sure to order just what is figured in the list below. My guess is that you will be charged the same price as you would for the greater amount of meat. Alternatively, you can ask that the rest of the meat be wrapped for you and then make yourself another sandwich with it the next day. Or just ask that three ounces of meat be put in the sandwich and the rest on top (to be used later). The deli has a scale right there. Since you know you have a special request, go early or late to avoid the crowd. Your order may not be filled if there are too many customers waiting in line. To complete your deli menu, order a diet drink and a piece of fruit. Stay away from deli potato salad, cole slaw, bean salad, and sweet pickles.

For quick reference, here are the calorie counts of typical deli food. You can see why you can't complete your menu from the deli counter:

Item	Quantity	Calories
Fresh fruit salad	1 cup	79
Gefilte	4 ounces	209
Pickled herring	2 ounces	126
Smoked salmon	4 ounces	200
Bagel	3-inch	165
Yeast donut	4-inch	170
Blueberry muffin	3-inch	125
Hoagie roll	1	390

Item	Quantity	Calories
Cream cheese	1 ounce	96
Potato salad	1/2 cup	124
Yogurt (fruit)	1 cup	245
Creamed cottage cheese	1 cup	240
Dill pickle	4-inch	15
Sour pickle	4-inch	14
Sweet gherkin pickle	3-inch	51
Pickle relish	1 tablespoon	21

Item	Quantity	Calories
Week 1		
Monday		
Bacon, lettuce, tomato sandwich	3 strips bacon	273
Tuesday		
Corned beef on rye	2 ounces meat	296
Wednesday		
Reuben	2 ounces meat	325
Thursday		
Lobster salad	4 ounces	280
Friday		
Turkey	5 ounces turkey	380
Week 2		
Monday		
Shrimp salad	4 ounces	250
Tuesday		
Pepper loaf and Swiss	3 ounces meat	
	1 ounce cheese	396
Wednesday		
Lox and bagel with onions and tomatoes	2 ounces lox	399
Thursday		
Pastrami	5 ounces	400
Friday		
Tuna salad	4 ounces	292

Restaurant Food Menus

Here I will give you a large selection of food items from various types of restaurants. I know that it is difficult to figure out what to eat and what to avoid. Maybe this short guide will help out. Choose soup or salad, one vegetable, and one entrée and try and do without dessert.

CHINESE RESTAURANT

MENU 1

Item	Quantity	Calories
Egg roll	1	139
Pork dumpling	1	48
Won ton soup	8 ounces	66
Won ton	1	41
Chicken cashew	1 cup	375
Sweet and sour pork	1 cup	343
Egg fried rice	½ cup	161

MENU 2

Fried shrimp	1 shrimp	86
Barbecued spare ribs	3 ribs	331
Egg flower soup	8 ounces	94
Beef and pea pods	1 cup	324
Shrimp in black bean sauce	1 cup	440
Steamed rice	½ cup	100
Soy sauce	1 tablespoon	8

MEXICAN RESTAURANT _____

MENU 1

Item	Quantity	Calories
Guacamole	¼ cup	85
Tortilla chips	1 chip	11
Black bean soup	6 ounces	204
Carne asada	4 ounces	307
Cheese enchilada	1	247
Paella	½ cup	250
Sopapillas	3-inch square	113
Bunuelos	1	226

MENU 2

Item	Quantity	Calories
Tomato chili dip	½ cup	54
Tortilla chip	1 chip	11
Gazpacho	6 ounces	183
Arroz con pollo	4 ounces	350
Chicken taco	1	175
Beef taco	1	204
Chile rellenos	1	127
Refried beans	¼ cup	120
Spanish rice	½ cup	150
Flan	½ cup	380

ITALIAN RESTAURANT

MENU 1

Item	Quantity	Calories
Melon and prosciutto	average serving	116
Fried mushrooms	4 pieces	199
Meat and spinach cannelloni	2 pieces	391
Ricotta cannelloni	2 pieces	358
Fettuccini Alfredo	1 cup	393
Spaghetti and meat sauce	1 cup	335
Stuffed squid	3 ounces	178
Zuppa inglese	average serving	372

MENU 2

Item	Quantity	Calories
Clams Casino	4 large clams	283
Minestrone soup	1 cup	151
Veal scaloppine	6 ounces	415
Veal parmesan	6 ounces	529
Tortellini in parsley and butter	12 pieces	294
Chicken Florentine	4 ounces	301
Zabaglione	½ cup	211

GREEK RESTAURANT

MENU 1

Item	Quantity	Calories
Bourekia	1 piece	96
Rice dolmades	1	46
Lamb dolmades	1	61
Marinated octopus	4 ounces	193
Lentil soup	8 ounces	238
Moussaka	2 3 × 4-inch pieces	539
Rice pilaf	¾ cup	29
Halva	2-inch piece	220

MENU 2

Item	Quantity	Calories
Lamb-stuffed cabbage	1 roll	163
Tyropites	1 piece	104
Tahini soup	8 ounces	186
Tomato feta salad	1 tomato	219
Lamb-stuffed green pepper	1 pepper	163
Veal avgolemono	5 ounces	470
Chicken Kakkinisto	4 ounces	304
Baklava	1 piece	400

FRENCH RESTAURANT

MENU 1

Item	Quantity	Calories
Salade de crabe farci	½ avocado	400
Marinated mushrooms	4 ounces	219
Pâté de campagne	½-ounce slice	267
Ham crêpe in cream sauce	1 crepe	156
Pistou	1 cup	365
Fondue de Gruyère with 1 slice bread	3½ ounces	489
Fruits de mer	4 ounces fish	277
Suprême de volaille cordon bleu	1 breast	346
Oeufs à la neige	average serving	343
Mousse sabayon	average serving	205

MENU 2

Item	Quantity	Calories
Shrimp cocktail	3 shrimp	330
Escargots Bourgogne	6 snails	418
Bisque de homard	1 cup	365
Cheese soufflé	1 cup	143
Coquilles Saint-Jacques	average serving	272
Coq au vin rouge	4 ounces	403
Asperges Hollandaise	6 spears	352
Pommes duchesse	1 potato	229
Éclair au chocolat	4-inch piece	367

GERMAN RESTAURANT

MENU 1

Item	Quantity	Calories
Tongue salad	½ cup	242
Pastry-wrapped sausages	1	243
Goulash soup	1 cup	312
Chicken Vienna	¼ pound	283
Sauerbraten	7 ounces	532
Sacher torte	4-inch piece	263

MENU 2

Item	Quantity	Calories
Pickled herring in sour cream	4 ounces	307
Grilled bratwurst	6 ounces	494
Sauerkraut kuchen	3-inch square	194
Wiener Schnitzel	2 cutlets	602
Pork loin roast with prunes and apples	4 ounces	451
Sweet and sour cabbage	1 cup	123
Spaetzle with butter	½ cup	98
Springerle	1	98
German chocolate torte	3-inch square	436

SEAFOOD RESTAURANT

MENU 1

Item	Quantity	Calories
Manhattan clam chowder	1 1/2 cups	122
Spinach bacon salad	2 cups	198
Thousand Island dressing	1 tablespoon	80
Broiled lobster tails	2 2-ounce tails	130
Fillet of sole amandine	6 ounces	508
Green beans	1/2 cup	13
Potatoes au gratin	1/2 cup	178
Hard French roll	1	80
Boston cream pie	1 serving	415

MENU 2

Item	Quantity	Calories
Chicken consommé	1 1/2 cups	33
Hearts of lettuce	1/4 head	18
Blue cheese dressing	1 tablespoon	94
Salmon steak	4 ounces	296
Fried shrimp	6 ounces	384
Peas and carrots	1/2 cup	46
French fries	10	137
Parker House roll	1	80
Chocolate cake	1 piece	550

STEAKHOUSE RESTAURANT

MENU 1

Item	Quantity	Calories
Crab cocktail	½ cup crab	89
Steak and lobster	8-ounce sirloin	470
	2-ounce tail	65
Steak Teriyaki	6 ounces	334
Filet mignon	8 ounces	468
Fresh peas	½ cup	82
Scalloped potatoes	½ cup	128
Apple pie	1 piece	404

MENU 2

Item	Quantity	Calories
T-bone steak	8 ounces	506
Prime rib, lean	8 ounces	565
Corn on the cob	1 ear	70
Baked potato	1	145
Orange sherbet	½ cup	130
Cheesecake	1 piece	525

5

Fast Food Substitution Menus

I do not think that it is possible for most Americans to give up fast food completely. During the past twenty years it has become a staple of our diet. We all end up grabbing something to eat at a fast food restaurant or driving through for a meal. What a shock this phenomenon would be to our ancestors. Enjoy yourself, but remember the "Rules of Eating" when having fast food.

Just one rule applies to eating fast food. Do not eat while you are driving. Drive to the park, the beach, or to any surroundings you enjoy. If possible, take the food out of the car and make a picnic of it. Keep a small basket in the car with plates, glasses, flatware, napkins, and a tablecloth. Then you are ready for any spur-of-the-moment "picnic." Remember that you must eat slowly. Don't be tempted to eat on the run. It's easy if you just plan your eating ahead of time.

The breakfast, lunch, and dinner menus in this chapter can be substituted for menus on the regular diet when necessary. But don't let the long lists of fried foods at fast food restaurants ruin or slow down your dieting effort. Try not to go to a fast food restaurant more than twice a week.

If you follow these fast food menus, you will not exceed your daily caloric allowance by much. If you order an additional item, you will go way over your allowance and the day after this indulgence you will be starving to try to catch up. Don't fall into this fast food trap.

As you read through the menus, it may not seem that you get much to eat, but each menu will satisfy your appetite. If you would like to order something else, just refer to the calorie chart for fast food restaurants to see if there are any other items that will fit into your daily allowance, but be careful in your substitutions.

In menus that include a salad bar, you should start with 2 cups of lettuce and then add onions, 3 ounces of tomatoes, cucumbers, radishes, celery, and bean sprouts. You can add the Bac-o-bits if you want, but you must remember that 1/4 ounce equals 29 calories. Calories do add up fast. Do not take any beans; they just add unnecessary calories. For dressing, I suggest that you carry your own diet dressing, which comes in 1-ounce packages containing only 4 calories each. By reducing the number of calories in the salad bar selection, you'll earn yourself a second helping. You will feel really full, but you won't be full of calories. Make sure to order a noncaloric beverage like herb tea, or bring your own diet soda with no caffeine and order a glass of ice.

Caution: These menus are not to be used more than twice per week.

Breakfast Menus

BREAKFAST MENU #1 AT MCDONALD'S

Egg McMuffin	352
Decaffeinated coffee	0
Total Calories	352

BREAKFAST MENU #2 AT MCDONALD'S

Hot cakes with butter and syrup	472
Decaffeinated coffee	0
Total Calories	472

BREAKFAST MENU #3 AT MCDONALD'S

Scrambled eggs	162
English muffin	186
Total Calories	348

If you decide to add something to your menu, just remember that the calories you add will put you way over your allowance for breakfast. As a reminder, here is the calorie count for the remainder of McDonald's breakfast items.

Hash brown potatoes	130
Pork sausage	184

BREAKFAST MENU #1 AT HARDEE'S

Biscuit with egg	383
Decaffeinated coffee	0
Total Calories	383

BREAKFAST MENU #2 AT HARDEE'S

Sausage biscuit with egg	521
Decaffeinated coffee	0
Total Calories	521

BREAKFAST MENU #3 AT HARDEE'S

Steak biscuit	419
Decaffeinated coffee	0
Total Calories	419

BREAKFAST MENU #1 AT JACK IN THE BOX

Breakfast Jack	301
Decaffeinated coffee	0
Total Calories	301

BREAKFAST MENU #2 AT JACK IN THE BOX

Double cheese omelet	423
Decaffeinated coffee	0
Total Calories	423

BREAKFAST MENU #3 AT JACK IN THE BOX

French toast breakfast	537
Decaffeinated coffee	0
Total Calories	537

Lunch Menus

LUNCH AT TACO BELL

Regular taco	159
Regular tostada	206
Iced tea	0
Total Calories	365

LUNCH AT BURGER KING

Whopper Jr.	369
Regular fries	209
Diet drink	3
Total Calories	581

LUNCH AT KENTUCKY FRIED CHICKEN

1 piece chicken, original recipe	199
Cole slaw	122
Mashed potatoes and gravy	86
Roll	61
Total Calories	468

LUNCH AT ARTHUR TREACHER'S FISH & CHIPS

1 piece fish	178
Chips	276
Coffee	0
Total Calories	454

LUNCH AT PIZZA HUT

2 slices standard pepperoni Thin 'n' Crispy	370
Salad Bar	
Lettuce, cucumber, bean sprouts, celery, Bac-o-bits, tomato	75
Total Calories	445

LUNCH AT GINO'S

Roast beef sandwich	413
Salad bar	75
Total Calories	488

Dinner Menus

DINNER AT FRIENDLY'S RESTAURANTS

Big beef with bread, butter	450
Vanilla ice cream with cake cone	248
Total Calories	698

DINNER AT LONG JOHN SILVER'S SEAFOOD SHOPPES

Shrimp with batter	269
Corn on the cob	174
Hush Puppies, 3 per order	153
Total Calories	596

DINNER AT MCDONALD'S

Quarter-pounder	418
Regular French fries	211
Total Calories	629

DINNER AT RUSTLER STEAK HOUSE

Filet mignon platter (do not eat roll and butter)	632
Salad bar	75
Total Calories	707

DINNER AT WENDY'S

Single hamburger	472
Chili	229
Total Calories	701

DINNER AT KENTUCKY FRIED CHICKEN

Drumstick and thigh dinner, original recipe	643
Corn	92
Total Calories	735

6

Beverages

You will find that each of these special melon drinks is a real pick-me-up. If you want to save the breakfast drink for your afternoon snack, do it. Also, if you're going to have a glass of wine in the afternoon, adding it to any of the "fruit shakes" makes a delicious drink.

Make a pitcher of these fruit beverages and then keep track of the portions and measure carefully. It is really handy to have the ice-cold beverages ready in the refrigerator. As a matter of fact, you will find your family begging you to let them have some, too.

Blackberry Melon Slush
   2 cups cantaloupe chunks
   2 cups blackberries
   3 cups diet 7-Up
   ¼ cup orange juice

Put the cantaloupe and the blackberries in a blender with the remaining ingredients. Whirl on frappé. Serve over ice.
Serves 6.

CALORIES: 40.7   CALCIUM: 20 mg.
PROTEIN: .9 gm.   SODIUM: 6.5 mg.
CARBOHYDRATE: 9.9 gm.   CHOLESTEROL: 0 mg.
FAT: .2 gm.

Melon Shake

2 cups cantaloupe chunks
1 cup orange juice
½ cup pineapple juice
½ cup grapefruit juice
3 packets lo-cal sweetener
1 tablespoon honey
1 cup water
10 ice cubes

Combine all the ingredients in a blender and whirl until smooth. *Serves 6.*

CALORIES: 54.8   CALCIUM: 17.2 mg.
PROTEIN: .9 gm.   SODIUM: 7.2 mg.
CARBOHYDRATE: 15 gm.   CHOLESTEROL: 0 mg.
FAT: .1 gm.

Melon Slush

½ cantaloupe
½ can frozen lemonade, thawed
1 quart diet 7-Up

Cut the cantaloupe into pieces and put in the blender. Turn blender on frappé and add the lemonade. Blend together and pour into a container. When ready to serve, put ⅔ cup of melon slush in a glass filled with ice. Fill glass with diet 7-Up. This mixture can also be frozen and makes a delicious warm weather treat. *Makes 6 cups.*

CALORIES: 41   CALCIUM: 38 mg.
PROTEIN: .9 gm.   SODIUM: 6.6 mg.
CARBOHYDRATE: 10.2 gm.   CHOLESTEROL: 0 mg.
FAT: .1 gm.

Orange Melon Juice

2 cups orange juice
½ cup pineapple juice
1 cup puree of cantaloupe
10 ice cubes

Put first three ingredients in a blender and then add the ice cubes.
Whirl on frappé. Serve chilled.
Serves 4.

CALORIES: 84.8   CALCIUM: 22.7 mg.
PROTEIN: 1.4 gm.   SODIUM: 10.8 mg.
CARBOHYDRATE: 20 gm.   CHOLESTEROL: 0 mg.
FAT: .4 gm.

Melon Julep

2 cups melon balls
2 tablespoons crushed mint leaves
1 tablespoon tangerine juice
1 packet lo-cal sweetener

Put the ingredients in a bowl. Cover and chill overnight. Serve cold.
You can also mix the ingredients in a blender and serve as a
beverage.
Serves 4.

CALORIES: 26.4   CALCIUM: 11 mg.
PROTEIN: .6 gm.   SODIUM: 9.7 mg.
CARBOHYDRATE: 6.4 gm.   CHOLESTEROL: 0 mg.
FAT: .1 gm.

7

Soups

On this diet, soup is your salvation. Since it really fills you up, you'll be happy to see that most of the meals begin with soup. The calories in these soups are usually negligible so if you're slightly overextended on the day's calories, have another cup of soup and then eat a little less of the entrée.

I always carry packets of lo-cal soup in my purse. No matter where you are, you can usually find a pot of hot water. Then when you get a sudden craving for food, you can satisfy it with a quick 10-calorie cup of soup. You will also find that it gives you a lift. You can purchase lo-cal soup packets in the grocery store. They come in small boxes with about ten packets in each box. Remember, you want the one with the fewest calories. Some of those soups contain 70 calories per packet. If there isn't a calorie count on the box, beware! Purchase only the soups that are between 10 and 16 calories per packet.

When those nasty fat cells are screaming "Food, food," you can hold them off with a cup of broth. You can have as much broth as you want. Believe me, your stomach will be full before you have reached even 40 calories. So while on this diet consider broth of 10 to 14 calories per cup free snacks.

Creamed Soup Base

¼ cup celery, sliced thin
⅓ cup onion, chopped
½ cup lo-cal chicken broth
2 tablespoons diet margarine
2 tablespoons flour
2 cups 2 percent milk

Cook the celery and onion in the chicken broth until limp. Put into a food processor and whirl until pureed. Meanwhile, melt the margarine in a saucepan and stir in the flour. Cook this mixture, called a roux, over medium heat for 3 minutes, stirring frequently. Pour the milk into the roux, stirring constantly with a whisk. Continue to stir until the sauce is thickened. Stir in the pureed vegetables and turn the heat down to simmer. Simmer 15 minutes. Put the soup through a strainer if you want it perfectly smooth.
Serves 6.

CALORIES: 80.2
PROTEIN: 4 gm.
CARBOHYDRATE: 8 gm.
FAT: 3.8 gm.

CALCIUM: 122.2 mg.
SODIUM: 117 mg.
CHOLESTEROL: 5 mg.

Apple Soup

1 apple
1 cup apple juice
⅓ cup orange juice
¼ cup sour cream
1 tablespoon honey
⅔ cup water
1 teaspoon lemon juice

Peel and core the apple, and dice it into small pieces. Combine the remaining ingredients and stir in the diced apple. Chill.
Serves 4.

CALORIES: 84.75
PROTEIN: 6.93 gm.
CARBOHYDRATE: 18.48 gm.
FAT: .53 gm.

CALCIUM: 25.79 mg.
SODIUM: 6.5 mg.
CHOLESTEROL: 18 mg.

Broccoli Bisque

1 recipe Creamed Soup Base
2 cups cut broccoli

Prepare 1 recipe of Creamed Soup Base according to the directions on page 79. Place the broccoli in the food processor and whirl until pureed. Stir the puree into the chowder base and heat through. Garnish with parsley flakes.
Serves 8.

CALORIES: 62.3
PROTEIN: 3.7 gm.
CARBOHYDRATE: 7.7 gm.
FAT: 2.9 gm.

CALCIUM: 125 mg.
SODIUM: 91 mg.
CHOLESTEROL: 3.7 mg.

Chicken Soup

1 cup water
1 chicken bouillon cube
1 teaspoon chopped chives
Dash pepper
1 tablespoon cooked chicken

Bring water to a boil and stir in and dissolve the bouillon cube. Add the remaining ingredients and heat through.
Serves 1.

CALORIES: 49
PROTEIN: 6.9 gm.
CARBOHYDRATE: 1.2 gm.
FAT: 1.7 gm.

CALCIUM: 2.2 mg.
SODIUM: 966 mg.
CHOLESTEROL: 12 mg.

Clam Chowder

1 tablespoon diet margarine
1/2 cup chopped onions
2 tomatoes, chopped
1/2 potato, peeled and diced
1 cup chicken broth
8 ounces tomato juice

1 tablespoon dry parsley flakes
1 clove garlic, minced
1 tablespoon catsup
1 teaspoon Bac-o-bits
1 teaspoon oregano
1/4 teaspoon thyme
1/4 teaspoon tarragon
1/4 teaspoon black pepper
2 cups water
12 ounces chopped clams

In a saucepan, melt the diet margarine and add the onions. Sauté until onions are clear. Stir in the tomatoes and sauté with the onions for 3 minutes. Add the diced potatoes and chicken broth. Cook over medium heat until the potatoes are done. Add the remaining ingredients. Bring the chowder to a boil, then turn down the heat and simmer for 30 minutes.
Serves 6.

CALORIES: 74
PROTEIN: 7.5 gm.
CARBOHYDRATE: 7 gm.
FAT: 3.6 gm.

CALCIUM: 53.3 mg.
SODIUM: 244 mg.
CHOLESTEROL: 90 mg.

Corn Chowder

1 recipe Creamed Soup Base
1 cup whole corn kernels
1/4 teaspoon dry mustard
1 tablespoon sherry
1 egg yolk, beaten

Prepare 1 recipe Creamed Soup Base according to the directions on page 79. Stir in the corn, dry mustard, and sherry. Whisk in the beaten egg yolk and heat through.
Serves 6.

CALORIES: 78.4
PROTEIN: 3.4 gm.
CARBOHYDRATE: 9.6 gm.
FAT: 3.5 gm.

CALCIUM: 64.2 mg.
SODIUM: 187 mg.
CHOLESTEROL: 45 mg.

Potato Soup

¼ cup onion, grated
3 cups chicken bouillon
1 cup water
1 cup 2 percent milk
1½ cups instant potato buds
White pepper
2 teaspoons chopped parsley
2 teaspoons minced chives

Combine the onions, bouillon, and water in a saucepan and bring to a boil. Remove from the heat and add ½ cup of the milk. Stir in the instant potato buds and whip several minutes. Stir in the remaining milk and the white pepper. Bring just to a boil over high heat. Remove from heat and chill. Stir in the parsley and sprinkle with chopped chives before serving. Serve cold or hot.
Serves 8.

CALORIES: 60.5
PROTEIN: 3.2 gm.
CARBOHYDRATE: 4.5 gm.
FAT: 1.8 gm.

CALCIUM: 48.4 mg.
SODIUM: 411 mg.
CHOLESTEROL: 1 mg.

Vegetable Soup

4 cups vegetable bouillon
1 carrot, julienne
½ cup chopped onion
¼ cup green beans, cut into 1-inch pieces
¼ cup tomato, diced
¼ cup sliced celery
1 tablespoon dry parsley flakes
1 bay leaf
3 peppercorns

Put the vegetable bouillon in a small stock pot. Bring to a boil. Drop in the prepared vegetables and the seasonings. Turn the heat down to simmer and cover. Simmer 35 minutes.
Serves 4.

CALORIES: 35.2
PROTEIN: 2 gm.
CARBOHYDRATE: 7.9 gm.
FAT: 1.1 gm.

CALCIUM: 24.3 mg.
SODIUM: 262 mg.
CHOLESTEROL: 0 mg.

Watercress Soup

1 recipe Creamed Soup Base
2 cups chopped watercress

Prepare 1 recipe Creamed Soup Base according to the directions on page 79. Heat the base through. Place 1 1/2 cups of chopped watercress into the food processor and puree. Stir into the soup base. Stir in the remaining 1/2 cup of chopped watercress and heat. *Serves 6.*

CALORIES: 88.2
PROTEIN: 29.8 gm.
CARBOHYDRATE: 9.3 gm.
FAT: 3.9 gm.

CALCIUM: 169.4 mg.
SODIUM: 132 mg.
CHOLESTEROL: 5 mg.

Wonton Soup

8 wonton skins
2 cups chicken bouillon
2 green onions, sliced
1 teaspoon soy sauce

Fold the wontons into triangles, sealing the edges with water. Bring the bouillon to a boil and add the green onions and the soy sauce. Drop the folded wontons into the soup and cook until the wontons are done. *Serves 4.*

CALORIES: 40
PROTEIN: 3 gm.
CARBOHYDRATE: 5 gm.
FAT: 2 gm.

CALCIUM: 20 mg.
SODIUM: 810 mg.
CHOLESTEROL: 0 mg.

Blueberry Melon Soup

1 recipe Cantaloupe Soup
1 cup frozen blueberries, crushed

Prepare 1 Cantaloupe Soup recipe according to directions below. Pour into a bowl. Add the blueberries. Chill. Serve in large wine glasses. *Serves 4*

CALORIES: 64
PROTEIN: 1.62 gm.
CARBOHYDRATE: 14.7 gm.
FAT: .15 gm.

CALCIUM: 58.96 mg.
SODIUM: 40 mg.
CHOLESTEROL: 37.8 mg.

Cantaloupe Soup

This recipe is so simple and delicious. It goes into the blender or food processor and comes out in seconds.

    ½ cantaloupe, peeled and diced
    ½ teaspoon lo-cal sweetener
    1 teaspoon honey
    ¼ cup orange juice
    1 teaspoon lemon juice
    ½ cup 2 percent milk
    ½ cup sour cream

Whirl the cantaloupe in the food processor (it should equal 1 cup). Pour out into a bowl. Add the remaining ingredients. Chill. Serve in large wine glasses.
Serves 4.

CALORIES: 44   CALCIUM: 49.96 mg.
PROTEIN: 1.62 gm.   SODIUM: 39 mg.
CARBOHYDRATE: 9.75 gm. CHOLESTEROL: 38 mg.
FAT: .15 gm.

Consommé with Melon

    1 10-ounce can consommé
    10 ounces water
    1 cup cantaloupe balls
    3 tablespoons chopped chives

Heat the consommé and the water together. Just before serving stir in the cantaloupe balls and the chopped chives. Sprinkle with fresh ground pepper.
Serves 4.

CALORIES: 17.6   CALCIUM: 5.5 mg.
PROTEIN: .3 gm.   SODIUM: 490 mg.
CARBOHYDRATE: 3 gm.   CHOLESTEROL: 0 mg.
FAT: Trace

Raspberry Melon Soup

1 recipe Cantaloupe Soup
1 cup frozen raspberries, crushed
½ cup sour cream

Prepare 1 recipe Cantaloupe Soup according to directions on page 84. Pour out into a bowl. Add the raspberries and the sour cream. Chill. Serve in large wine glasses.
Serves 4.

CALORIES: 64
PROTEIN: 1.9 gm.
CARBOHYDRATE: 14.7 gm.
FAT: .15 gm.

CALCIUM: 58.9 mg.
SODIUM: 40 mg.
CHOLESTEROL: 38 mg.

Maryland Crab Soup

8 ounces crabmeat
¼ cup chopped onion
1 tablespoon chopped green pepper
1 clove garlic, minced
1 bay leaf
¼ teaspoon thyme
2 cups tomato juice
1 cup chicken bouillon
1 tablespoon parsley, minced
¼ teaspoon seafood seasoning
¼ teaspoon Worcestershire sauce
2 tablespoons sherry

Combine all the ingredients in a saucepan and bring to a boil. Turn down the heat and simmer for 30 minutes. Serve hot.
Serves 4.

CALORIES: 96.2
PROTEIN: 11.7 gm.
CARBOHYDRATE: 6.1 gm.
FAT: 2.6 gm.

CALCIUM: 41.4 mg.
SODIUM: 250 mg.
CHOLESTEROL: 90 mg.

8

Salads

Have you ever asked the chronic dieter what he or she is eating? The answer is always "Lots of salad."

One of the Annapolis Diet's greatest assets is its wide selection of salads. I have put a variety of ingredients in these salads to make them just a bit more exciting. The fruit and vegetable combinations and the spicy dressings should keep you interested. But the best aspect of salad is that it adds volume to the meal and helps to fill the stomach fast. The brain gets a signal that you are full and you have eaten only about 50 calories. What more could the serious dieter ask for?

Every time you go to the store, buy two extra heads of lettuce. Clean them and break each head into bite-size pieces. Store in a plastic bag. (Hint: If you wash the lettuce in lukewarm water, drain it until it is just moist, and then put it in the plastic bag, the lettuce will not turn brown for at least three or four days.) Now you can have a salad anytime you wish. People who are overweight will usually reach for something convenient when they are hungry, so snack foods and sweets are their downfall because they are always handy.

Why shouldn't you reach for salad instead? Just make it easy for yourself and you'll find yourself "grabbing for greens." When you purchase the diet dressings, be sure you look at the calorie count on the bottles; you'll be amazed at how high some of them are. See if you can find a variety that is made without oil. It's usually the lowest in calories, with around 10 to 15 calories per serving. Just remember to shop with caution and read the labels.

Do you realize that in order to obtain the 270 calories found in a candy bar, you would have to consume twelve heads of Boston lettuce? When I lectured the midshipmen at the Naval Academy on dieting, I brought about twenty food items with me. I weighed and measured the items so that each was equal to 150 calories. The lettuce took nearly half the table; the candy bar had to cut into a smaller piece; the eleven potato chips were barely noticeable; and the cucumbers, cauliflower, and broccoli occupied the other half of the table. My point to the mids was this: Eat all that you want, but make it the right stuff.

At the Academy, a jar of peanut butter is always placed on the dining tables just in case the midshipmen don't like the food being served. It is common to see midshipmen walking out of the dining hall carrying a jar of peanut butter. So as part of my lecture to the mids, I measured out 150 calories of peanut butter. It was less than 2 tablespoons, a shockingly scant quantity when placed next to the lettuce! I then told them what an old acquaintance of mine had told me many years ago: The only place you should put peanut butter is on your face as a cream, *NEVER* in your mouth. Think of all the foodstuffs that should be used for the skin instead of the stomach!

The moral to this story is that lettuce is a free treat on any diet. If you've got to have that crunch in your mouth, make it lettuce instead of a potato chip. Rather, make it four bowls of lettuce with all the vinegar you want.

Bibb Salad

    1 tablespoon lemon juice
    3 tablespoons diet mayonnaise
    3 tablespoons orange juice
    1 cup seedless grapes
    1 orange, sliced
    1 apple, sliced
    2 heads Bibb lettuce
    2 slices lo-cal bacon, chopped

Place the lemon juice, diet mayonnaise, and orange juice into a salad bowl and whisk. Stir in the seedless grapes, the sliced orange, and the sliced apple. Toss with the dressing. Break the lettuce into bite-size pieces. Mix together. Sprinkle with chopped bacon that has been cooked until it is very crisp.
Serves 8.

CALORIES: 56.1   CALCIUM: 26.7 mg.
PROTEIN: 1.3 gm.   SODIUM: 25 mg.
CARBOHYDRATE: 9.5 gm.   CHOLESTEROL: 10 mg.
FAT: 1.7 gm.

Broccoli Salad

    1 cup bean sprouts
    2 cups chopped broccoli
    ¼ cup cauliflower, broken into flowerets
    ½ cup hearts of Romaine
    ¼ cup chopped green onion tops
    1 tablespoon watercress, sliced
    1 ounce diet Italian dressing

Clean and prepare the vegetables and place in a bowl. Toss with diet Italian dressing. Place in the refrigerator and chill 2 hours.
Serves 4.

CALORIES: 43   CALCIUM: 64.6 mg.
PROTEIN: 4 gm.   SODIUM: 91 mg.
CARBOHYDRATE: 6.8 gm.   CHOLESTEROL: 0 mg.
FAT: .4 gm.

Cabbage Salad

1 head cabbage, shredded
1 red onion, sliced
½ green pepper, sliced
2 carrots, grated
¼ cup red wine vinegar
1 teaspoon lo-cal sweetener
½ teaspoon dry mustard
½ teaspoon celery seed
1 cup water

In a large mixing bowl, combine the cabbage, red onion, green pepper, and carrots. In small bowl, beat the red wine vinegar, lo-cal sweetener, dry mustard, celery seed, and water. Pour the dressing over the cabbage and vegetable mixture. Toss together. Cover and chill overnight.
Serves 6.

CALORIES: 42
PROTEIN: 1.9 gm.
CARBOHYDRATE: 9.8 gm.
FAT: .2 gm.

CALCIUM: 63.3 mg.
SODIUM: 32 mg.
CHOLESTEROL: 0 mg.

Chef's Salad

½ head Romaine lettuce
1 cup chicory, chopped
1 head Boston lettuce
¾ ounce Swiss cheese, grated
¼ cup bean sprouts
¼ cup mushrooms, sliced
1 ounce blue cheese, crumbled
1 tomato, thinly sliced
1½ ounces Canadian bacon, julienne
¼ cup chopped cauliflower
1 ounce chicken, diced

Break the lettuce into bite-size pieces. In a large salad bowl toss all the ingredients together. Chill. Serve with diet salad dressing.
Serves 4.

CALORIES: 124
PROTEIN: 8.78 gm.
CARBOHYDRATE: 6.38 gm.
FAT: 7.25 gm.

CALCIUM: 161.5 mg.
SODIUM: 252 mg.
CHOLESTEROL: 38 mg.

Cucumber Salad

2 cucumbers, sliced
2 tomatoes, sliced
1 red onion, sliced
Fresh ground pepper
½ ounce diet Italian dressing
2 tablespoons red wine vinegar
1 teaspoon lemon juice
1 teaspoon oregano

Place the cucumbers, tomatoes, and red onion in layers in a glass bowl. In small bowl blend the pepper, diet Italian dressing, red wine vinegar, lemon juice, and oregano. Pour over the vegetables. Place in the refrigerator and marinate for 3 to 4 hours before serving. *Serves 4.*

CALORIES: 47.25
PROTEIN: 1.39 gm.
CARBOHYDRATE: 8.4 gm.
FAT: .3 gm.

CALCIUM: 30.4 mg.
SODIUM: 39 mg.
CHOLESTEROL: 0 mg.

Duck Salad

⅓ cup crushed pineapple, drained
¼ cup white vinegar
2 tablespoons beef bouillon
3 tablespoons chopped onion
1 teaspoon curry powder
8 lychee nuts
1 head Boston lettuce
8 ounces cooked duck meat

Put the drained crushed pineapple into a mixing bowl and add the vinegar, bouillon, onion, curry powder, and the lychee nuts. Blend well. Break the lettuce into bite-size pieces and put on a serving platter. Put the duck meat on the lettuce and spoon the pineapple dressing over that. *Serves 2.*

CALORIES: 236
PROTEIN: 15.4 gm.
CARBOHYDRATE: 19 gm.
FAT: 10.8 gm.

CALCIUM: 41.1 mg.
SODIUM: 125 mg.
CHOLESTEROL: 92 mg.

Endive Salad

1 bunch endive, broken into bite-size pieces
1 head Boston lettuce, broken into bite-size pieces
1/2 cup chopped watercress
1 sliced zucchini

Clean the ingredients and toss in a large mixing bowl. Serve chilled with diet dressing.
Serves 4.

CALORIES: 19.2
PROTEIN: 1.7 gm.
CARBOHYDRATE: 3.3 gm.
FAT: .6 gm.

CALCIUM: 54.5 mg.
SODIUM: 12 mg.
CHOLESTEROL: 0 mg.

Italian Salad

1 head Romaine lettuce
1/2 cup Chinese parsley, chopped
1/2 cup zucchini, sliced
1 tomato, chopped
4 radishes, sliced
1/2 ounce Provolone cheese, grated
1 ounce salami, minced
1 red onion, sliced
1 clove garlic, minced
2 anchovy fillets, mashed

Clean the lettuce and vegetables. Break the lettuce into bite-size pieces. Toss all the ingredients together in a large salad bowl. Chill. Serve with diet dressing.
Serves 4.

CALORIES: 65.1
PROTEIN: 8 gm.
CARBOHYDRATE: 5.9 gm.
FAT: 2.4 gm.

CALCIUM: 50.6 mg.
SODIUM: 40 mg.
CHOLESTEROL: 9 mg.

Lettuce Hearts

    ½ heart iceberg lettuce
    Diet salad dressing
    Black pepper

Cut the lettuce into 4 wedges. Place on a serving platter. Serve with diet dressing and freshly ground black pepper.
Serves 4.

CALORIES: 17   CALCIUM: 27 mg.
PROTEIN: 1.2 gm.   SODIUM: 6 mg.
CARBOHYDRATE: 3.2 gm.   CHOLESTEROL: 0 mg.
FAT: .1 gm.

Red-Leaf Lettuce Salad

    1 head red-leaf lettuce, broken into bite-size pieces
    ¼ cup cucumber, sliced
    ½ cup green beans, sliced thin
    ½ cantaloupe, cut into chunks

Toss all the ingredients together in a large salad bowl. Serve with diet dressing.
Serves 4.

CALORIES: 28   CALCIUM: 28.75 mg.
PROTEIN: .98 gm.   SODIUM: 6.4 mg.
CARBOHYDRATE: 3.15 gm.   CHOLESTEROL: 0 mg.
FAT: .13 gm.

Tossed Romaine Salad

    1 head Romaine lettuce
    6 green onions, sliced
    4 radishes, sliced
    ¼ cup chopped watercress
    ¼ teaspoon coarse pepper
    4 large mushrooms, sliced

In a mixing bowl break the lettuce into bite-size pieces. Toss with the remaining ingredients and chill. Serve with diet salad dressing.
Serves 4.

CALORIES: 34.75   CALCIUM: 68.5 mg.
PROTEIN: 2.38 gm.   SODIUM: 11 mg.
CARBOHYDRATE: 6.73 gm.   CHOLESTEROL: 0 mg.
FAT: .38 gm.

Tuna Salad in Tomato Cups

    4 tomatoes
    7½ ounces tuna, packed in water
    ½ cup chopped green onion
    2 hard-cooked eggs, chopped
    ¼ cup sliced sweet pickles
    4 ounces diet Thousand Island dressing
    Lettuce
    Lemon twists

Cut the tops from the tomatoes and wash. Scoop out the center of each tomato, forming a cup. Reserve tomato pulp. In a mixing bowl place the tuna, onion, hard-cooked eggs, pickles, and tomato pulp. Pour in the Thousand Island dressing. Blend well. Fill the tomato cups and serve on a platter in a bed of lettuce. Garnish with lemon twists.

Serves 4.

CALORIES: 152.5
PROTEIN: 18.8 gm.
CARBOHYDRATE: 10.2 gm.
FAT: 3.5 gm.

CALCIUM: 51.5 mg.
SODIUM: 265 mg.
CHOLESTEROL: 174 mg.

Cabbage Melon Salad

    3 packets lo-cal sweetener
    ¼ cup rice wine vinegar
    ½ teaspoon Oriental sesame oil
    6 cups shredded cabbage
    ¼ teaspoon minced fresh ginger
    ⅛ teaspoon minced fresh garlic
    3 tablespoons sliced green onion tops
    1 cup cantaloupe balls

In a mixing bowl combine the sweetener, rice wine vinegar, and sesame oil. Put the cabbage in the bowl and toss with the dressing. Sprinkle with the ginger, garlic, and onion tops. Add the cantaloupe balls. Toss gently until mixed. Chill 1 hour before serving.

Serves 6.

CALORIES: 42
PROTEIN: 1.9 gm.
CARBOHYDRATE: 9.8 gm.
FAT: .2 gm.

CALCIUM: 63.3 mg.
SODIUM: 18 mg.
CHOLESTEROL: 0 mg.

Spinach Melon Salad

1 bunch straw mushrooms
1/2 cup chicken bouillon
Pinch dried red pepper flakes
1/2 cup finely chopped onion
2 tablespoons light soy sauce
1/4 cup diet Russian dressing
8 cups fresh spinach leaves
1 cup boiling water
1 teaspoon lemon juice
2 cups cantaloupe balls
1 tablespoon peanuts

Clean and trim the straw mushrooms. Combine in a heavy skillet with the chicken bouillon. Simmer uncovered for 5 minutes. Remove from heat. Lift the mushrooms out of the liquid and discard liquid. Cool. In a saucepan put the red pepper flakes, onion, soy sauce, and Russian dressing. Place over low heat and stir until smooth. Meanwhile, clean the spinach and place in a colander. Pour boiling water over the spinach leaves. Put the spinach and mushrooms in a large dish towel and ring them dry. Then put the spinach and mushrooms in a serving bowl and sprinkle with 1 teaspoon lemon juice. Add the cantaloupe balls and peanuts and toss. Pour a little dressing over the salad just to moisten. Pass remaining dressing.
Serves 6.

CALORIES: 58.6
PROTEIN: 14.8 gm.
CARBOHYDRATE: 20.2 gm.
FAT: 8.7 gm.

CALCIUM: 221.5 mg.
SODIUM: 561 mg.
CHOLESTEROL: 0 mg.

Marinated Broccoli

1 bunch fresh broccoli
3/4 cup cider vinegar
2 tablespoons cold water
1/4 cup beef bouillon
1 packet lo-cal sweetener
1/2 teaspoon lemon peel

2 teaspoons dillseeds
1/4 teaspoon pepper
1/2 teaspoon minced garlic
4 ripe olives
3 tablespoons chopped pimento

Wash the broccoli and cut up. Peel the stems. Cut the broccoli into serving-size pieces. Place in a serving dish. Meanwhile, put the vinegar, water, bouillon, lo-cal sweetener, lemon peel, and spices into a mixing bowl and whisk the ingredients together. Pour the dressing over the broccoli and garnish with the sliced olives and the pimento.
Serves 6.

CALORIES: 26
PROTEIN: 1.5 gm.
CARBOHYDRATE: 2.6 gm.
FAT: .4 gm.

CALCIUM: 41.2 mg.
SODIUM: 60 mg.
CHOLESTEROL: 0 mg.

German Salad

Dressing:

2 tablespoons lemon juice
1/4 cup cider vinegar
3 tablespoons applesauce
1/2 teaspoon dry mustard
2 tablespoons parsley
Pinch garlic powder

2 apples, sliced
2 cups shredded green cabbage
1/4 cup shredded red cabbage
1 small onion, sliced
1/4 head lettuce

Blend the dressing ingredients in a mixing bowl. Toss the apples, cabbage, and onion together in a salad bowl and add to the dressing. Marinate 2 hours. Serve drained on a bed of lettuce.
Serves 4.

CALORIES: 81.8
PROTEIN: 1.17 gm.
CARBOHYDRATE: 20 gm.
FAT: .65 gm.

CALCIUM: 48 mg.
SODIUM: 14 mg.
CHOLESTEROL: 0 mg.

Shrimp Louis

8 ounces cooked shrimp, chopped
1 cup celery, sliced
2 tablespoons green onion tops, sliced
1/8 teaspoon pepper
1/4 cup diet mayonnaise
2 teaspoons lemon juice
4 cups shredded lettuce
1 tomato, sliced
1 hard-cooked egg, chopped

In a mixing bowl toss the shrimp, celery, green onion tops, and pepper with the mayonnaise and lemon juice. Place the shredded lettuce on serving plates and top with the shrimp mixture. Place the tomato slices and hard-cooked egg on each plate as garnish. *Serves 4.*

CALORIES: 104.5
PROTEIN: 13.25 gm.
CARBOHYDRATE: 7.2 gm.
FAT: 2.12 gm.

CALCIUM: 98.75 mg.
SODIUM: 78 mg.
CHOLESTEROL: 117 mg.

Tostada Salad

4 corn tortillas
1/4 pound lean ground beef
1/2 cup chopped onion
1 teaspoon chili powder
1 clove garlic, pressed
1/4 teaspoon pepper
Dash red pepper
1/2 teaspoon Worcestershire sauce
1 cup shredded lettuce
1 cup chopped tomatoes
4 tablespoons sour cream
4 teaspoons chili sauce
2 ounces Cheddar cheese, grated
1/2 cup sliced green onion tops

Toast the tortillas on a baking sheet in the oven set at 400 degrees. Toast on one side for 6 minutes, then turn over to the other side and bake an additional 5 minutes until the shells are crisp.

Meanwhile, in a heavy skillet over medium heat, sauté the ground beef with 2 tablespoons of the onion. Stir in the chili powder, pressed garlic, pepper, red pepper, and Worcestershire sauce. Simmer until the ground beef and spices are well blended.

To assemble, place one tortilla on each serving platter. Divide the meat mixture into 4 equal portions and place on each tortilla. Top each of the tostadas with lettuce, tomatoes, the remaining onions, sour cream, hot chili sauce, and cheese. Serve hot, sprinkled with the green onion.

Serves 4.

CALORIES: 180.38   CALCIUM: 234.5 mg.
PROTEIN: 12.5 gm.   SODIUM: 306 mg.
CARBOHYDRATE: 16.39 gm.   CHOLESTEROL: 68 mg.
FAT: 9.23 gm.

Greek Salad

2 ounces Feta cheese
1 tablespoon lemon juice
Dash pepper
3 tablespoons beef bouillon
1 teaspoon wine vinegar
1 teaspoon oregano
2 cucumbers, sliced thinly
2 onions, sliced into rings
4 cups fresh spinach leaves
1 tablespoon minced Chinese parsley

Place 1 ounce of the Feta cheese in a food processor fitted with a steel blade. Add the lemon juice, pepper, bouillon, wine vinegar, and oregano. Whirl until well blended. In a mixing bowl, place the cucumbers, onions, remaining ounce of Feta cheese, spinach leaves, and Chinese parsley. Pour the dressing over the salad. Chill in the refrigerator for at least 1 hour.

Serves 4.

CALORIES: 55.3   CALCIUM: 190.5 mg.
PROTEIN: 6.4 gm.   SODIUM: 920 mg.
CARBOHYDRATE: 7.68 gm.   CHOLESTEROL: 64 mg.
FAT: 3.9 gm.

9

Salad Dressings

Salad dressings are hard to give up. The well-intentioned dieter often goes to the salad buffet and leaves the beans, croutons, and cheese, but adds 800 calories by topping his or her low-calorie salad with regular blue cheese dressing. Learn to use wine vinegar or tarragon vinegar on your salad and nothing else. It really is refreshing, and you'll never have that "ucky" thick oily taste in your mouth.

You can buy delicious low-calorie dressings today. You can even mix them together. Diet cucumber with a little diet French is great. Or combine diet blue cheese and diet Russian; you'll love it. It's important to experiment. Carry packets of diet dressing in your purse or your pocket for emergency situations.

The diet dressing recipes in this chapter are quick and easy to make. It's important to top your salad with something you know you'll like, so keep these dressings handy. You can increase the quantity and store the dressings in glass jars in the refrigerator. They will keep several weeks. Besides, it's fun to have your very own homemade selections.

The calculations for the nutritious contents of these salad dressing recipes is for the entire recipe. So if you use only 1 or 2 tablespoons you can see how few calories it really is! All you have to remember is that there are sixteen tablespoons per cup.

Creamy Cucumber Dressing

3 calories per tablespoon

> 2 packets lo-cal sweetener
> 3 tablespoons plain yogurt
> 1/4 cup minced cucumber, seeds removed
> 1 teaspoon red wine vinegar
> 1 tablespoon minced green onion
> 1/4 cup chicken bouillon
> 1/4 teaspoon crushed basil
> Dash white pepper

In a mixing bowl stir the lo-cal sweetener into the yogurt. Add the remaining ingredients and mix well. Chill in a covered glass jar.
Makes 3/4 cup of dressing.

CALORIES: 36.9
PROTEIN: 2.6 gm.
CARBOHYDRATE: 8.4 gm.
FAT: .75 gm.

CALCIUM: 65.2 mg.
SODIUM: 206.7 mg.
CHOLESTEROL: 3 mg.

Pineapple Curry Dressing

5.8 calories per tablespoon

This is great when served with duck or chicken salad.

> 1/4 cup pineapple juice
> 2 teaspoons white wine vinegar
> 1/4 cup beef bouillon
> 1 teaspoon curry powder
> 1 tablespoon minced green onion
> 1 packet lo-cal sweetener
> 1 teaspoon rose water

Put all the ingredients in a mixing bowl and blend. Chill in the refrigerator before serving.
Makes 1/2 cup.

CALORIES: 46.4
PROTEIN: 1.5 gm.
CARBOHYDRATE: 10 gm.
FAT: .08 gm.

CALCIUM: 11.5 mg.
SODIUM: 195.2 mg.
CHOLESTEROL: 0 mg.

Apple Salad Dressing
5.6 calories per tablespoon

Great served with sliced red and green cabbage.

    2 tablespoons lemon juice
    2 teaspoons apple juice
    1/4 cup cider vinegar
    2 tablespoons applesauce
    1/2 teaspoon dry mustard
    1 tablespoon minced parsley
    Pinch garlic powder
    3 tablespoons beef bouillon

Place all the ingredients in a mixing bowl and blend well.
Makes 1/2 cup dressing.

CALORIES: 44.9
PROTEIN: .98 gm.
CARBOHYDRATE: 23.1 gm.
FAT: .06 gm.

CALCIUM: 5 mg.
SODIUM: 100 mg.
CHOLESTEROL: 0 mg.

Diet Caesar Dressing
11.2 calories per tablespoon

    2 anchovies
    Milk
    1 coddled egg
    1 tablespoon lemon juice
    2 tablespoons red wine vinegar
    2 cloves garlic, minced
    1/4 cup beef bouillon
    1/8 teaspoon black pepper
    1 teaspoon Worcestershire sauce
    1 tablespoon grated Parmesan cheese
    Romaine leaves

Put the anchovies in a bowl with enough milk to cover them and marinate for 20 minutes. Remove and pat dry. Discard the milk. Mash the anchovies with the back of a fork in a salad bowl. Beat in the coddled egg. Add the remaining ingredients and pour over fresh Romaine lettuce leaves that have been left whole.

Makes 2/3 cup.

CALORIES: 135
PROTEIN: 11.2 gm.
CARBOHYDRATE: 4.6 gm.
FAT: 8 gm.

CALCIUM: 114 mg.
SODIUM: 320 mg.
CHOLESTEROL: 262 mg.

Seafood Salad Dressing

9.1 calories per tablespoon

> 1/4 cup plain yogurt
> 1 tablespoon minced green onion tops
> 1/4 teaspoon minced tarragon leaves
> 1/4 teaspoon dry mustard
> 1/2 teaspoon seafood seasoning
> 1 tablespoon diet mayonnaise
> Dash white pepper
> 1 tablespoon minced gherkins
> 2 teaspoons fresh lemon juice
> 1 teaspoon minced Chinese parsley
> 1 teaspoon capers

Blend the ingredients in a mixing bowl. Chill several hours or overnight before serving.

Makes 1/2 cup.

CALORIES: 73.3
PROTEIN: 2.5 gm.
CARBOHYDRATE: 13.2 gm.
FAT: 3 gm.

CALCIUM: 79.2 mg.
SODIUM: 50.8 mg.
CHOLESTEROL: 0 mg.

Red Pepper Dressing
7.9 calories per tablespoon

Beware, it's hot! This is great on fresh spinach leaves or cabbage.
Try it on curly endive for even more heat.

- 1/2 cup chicken broth
- 1/8 teaspoon dried red pepper flakes
- 2 tablespoons diet Russian dressing
- 1 teaspoon light soy sauce
- 2 tablespoons minced green onion tops
- 1/4 teaspoon minced garlic
- 1/2 teaspoon bruised rosemary

Blend the ingredients and chill.
Makes 1/2 cup.

CALORIES: 63.6
PROTEIN: 2 gm.
CARBOHYDRATE: 13.3 gm.
FAT: 4 gm.

CALCIUM: 17.3 mg.
SODIUM: 838 mg.
CHOLESTEROL: 0 mg.

Spicy Vinaigrette
4.7 calories per tablespoon

- 2 ounces diet Italian dressing
- 2 tablespoons red wine vinegar
- 1 packet lo-cal sweetener
- 2 tablespoons minced chives
- 1 clove garlic, minced
- 1/8 teaspoon crushed pepper
- 1 teaspoon oregano

Put the ingredients into a jar with a tight-fitting lid. Shake. Chill
before serving.
Makes 1/2 cup.

CALORIES: 38
PROTEIN: .2 gm.
CARBOHYDRATE: .6 gm.
FAT: 0 gm.

CALCIUM: 0 mg.
SODIUM: 473 mg.
CHOLESTEROL: 0 mg.

Low Calorie Blue Cheese Dressing
6.1 calories per tablespoon
- 1/4 cup diet blue cheese dressing
- 1/4 cup diet Italian dressing
- 1 tablespoon blue cheese
- 1 teaspoon white wine vinegar
- 1 teaspoon dry mustard
- 1 tablespoon yogurt

Put the ingredients in a small mixing bowl and blend, using a whisk.

Makes 1/2 cup.

CALORIES: 48.8
PROTEIN: .8 gm.
CARBOHYDRATE: 1 gm.
FAT: .7 gm.

CALCIUM: 21.5 mg.
SODIUM: 1,156 mg.
CHOLESTEROL: 0 mg.

Rice Wine Dressing
6.6 calories per tablespoon
- 3 packets lo-cal sweetener
- 1/4 cup rice wine vinegar
- 1 tablespoon chicken broth
- 1/2 teaspoon Oriental sesame oil
- 1/4 teaspoon light soy sauce
- 3 tablespoons sliced green onion tops
- 1/4 teaspoon minced fresh ginger
- 1/8 teaspoon minced garlic

Put ingredients into a mixing bowl and blend.

Makes 1/3 cup.

CALORIES: 33
PROTEIN: .3 gm.
CARBOHYDRATE: 2.2 gm.
FAT: 2.1 gm.

CALCIUM: 6 mg.
SODIUM: 109 mg.
CHOLESTEROL: 0 mg.

Fresh Lime Dressing
4 calories per tablespoon
>   ¼ cup beef broth
>   2 tablespoons fresh-squeezed lime juice
>   ½ teaspoon grated lime peel
>   Dash black pepper
>   ½ teaspoon Dijon mustard
>   ¼ teaspoon basil leaves
>   ¼ teaspoon tarragon leaves

Combine all the ingredients and blend.
Makes ⅓ cup.

CALORIES: 20.5
PROTEIN: 1.5 gm.
CARBOHYDRATE: 3.3 gm.
FAT: .1 gm.

CALCIUM: 5 mg.
SODIUM: 228 mg.
CHOLESTEROL: 0 mg.

Honey Dressing
12.5 calories per tablespoon

This is delicious when served with fresh fruit.
>   1/4 cup orange juice
>   1 teaspoon clover honey
>   Dash allspice
>   ½ teaspoon orange flower water

Put ingredients into a small mixing bowl and blend with a fork.
Makes ¼ cup.

CALORIES: 50.3
PROTEIN: .8 gm.
CARBOHYDRATE: 14.2 gm.
FAT: .1 gm.

CALCIUM: 7.2 mg.
SODIUM: .8 mg.
CHOLESTEROL: 0 mg.

10

Breads

American cuisine is almost centered around bread. In a restaurant, for instance, you are escorted to your table. You sit down and are handed the menu. Everyone is so helpful and polite. Then what happens before you can say a word? They bring a basket full of hot fresh bread. If that's not enough, they also put a bowl full of sweet delicious butter right in front of you. All of this happens before the no-calorie water arrives! I just die! It takes every bit of will power I possess not to eat every last slice of that white, rye, wheat, and pumpernickel before they even take my order! Have you ever devoured the bread and butter so that by the time the waiter comes to take your order, you are ready to ask for the check? Bread is a hard food to give up.

The first thing most people tell you when dieting is that you've got to give up bread. That is simply not true. Slender people eat bread. When you are dieting you just need to eat *less* bread and be sure it is thin-sliced—no more than 40 calories per slice. Make your sandwiches open-faced and you will save 40 calories, but you'll still get your sandwiches.

When dieting, just remember to add the 40 calories to your caloric intake for the day, and if you come in under 900 or 1,200 calories (depending on which plan you are following), you can have that slice of bread. If not, save the bread and have it for toast at breakfast the next day.

Chive Biscuits

    1 cup biscuit mix
    ¼ cup water
    3 tablespoons chopped chives
    6 drops liquid hot pepper seasoning
    2 teaspoons parsley flakes

Mix all the ingredients in a mixing bowl. Do not overbeat. Roll out dough ½-inch thick on a floured surface and cut into 1-inch rounds. Makes 16 1-inch biscuits.
Serves 8.

CALORIES: 64.6   CALCIUM: 6.4 mg.
PROTEIN: 1.4 gm.   SODIUM: 260 mg.
CARBOHYDRATE: 10.5 gm. CHOLESTEROL: 8 mg.
FAT: 1.9 gm.

French Toast

    1 egg
    2 tablespoons 2 percent milk
    ¼ teaspoon cinnamon
    ⅛ cup water
    2 slices diet (thin-sliced) bread
    Vegetable cooking spray

In a small mixing bowl, beat together the egg, milk, and cinnamon. Beat in the water. Quickly dip the bread slices into the egg mixture. Meanwhile, spray a skillet with vegetable cooking spray and heat the pan over medium heat. Place the egg-dipped bread slices in the heated pan. Turn the toast when lightly browned and toast the other side. Remove from the pan and place on a serving platter. Serve with diet maple syrup.
Serves 1.

CALORIES: 164   CALCIUM: 63.25 mg.
PROTEIN: 7.82 gm.   SODIUM: 170 mg.
CARBOHYDRATE: 13 gm.   CHOLESTEROL: 257 mg.
FAT: 7.5 gm.

Garlic Bread

4 slices very thin white bread
3 teaspoons diet margarine
Pinch garlic powder
1 teaspoon dried parsley flakes
Dash paprika
1/2 ounce Parmesan cheese

Place the bread slices on a baking sheet and spread with the margarine. Sprinkle with the garlic powder and parsley flakes. Dust with paprika and sprinkle with the Parmesan cheese.
Serves 6.

CALORIES: 66
PROTEIN: 3.2 gm.
CARBOHYDRATE: 3 gm.
FAT: 3.5 gm.

CALCIUM: 102 mg.
SODIUM: 37 mg.
CHOLESTEROL: 2 mg.

Garlic Sticks

1 tablespoon diet margarine, melted
2 cloves minced garlic
2 tablespoons minced parsley
4 slices very thin white bread

Mix the diet margarine, garlic, and parsley. Cut the bread slices into 1-inch strips. Spread the margarine mixture over each strip. Bake 10 minutes or until browned in an oven set at 475 degrees.
Serves 4.

CALORIES: 56.5
PROTEIN: 2.5 gm.
CARBOHYDRATE: 12.8 gm.
FAT: 6.6 gm.

CALCIUM: 23.9 mg.
SODIUM: 5 mg.
CHOLESTEROL: 0 mg.

Diet Pancakes

    4 tablespoons lo-cal pancake mix
    1 cup cold water
    Vegetable cooking spray

Place the pancake mix in a small mixing bowl. Using a whisk, beat in the cold water. Beat until smooth, but do not overbeat. Heat over medium high heat a skillet that has been sprayed with vegetable cooking spray. Pour the batter in the skillet, forming 3 4-inch pancakes. Cook until bubbles form on the top of pancakes, then turn. Cook until golden brown.
Serves 1 person 3 pancakes.

VARIATION: For Blueberry Pancakes, add 2 tablespoons drained blueberries.

CALORIES: 140
PROTEIN: 15 gm.
CARBOHYDRATE: 14.2 gm.
FAT: 2.2 gm.

CALCIUM: 15 mg.
SODIUM: 183 mg.
CHOLESTEROL: 114 mg.

11

Sandwich Fillings

When you "brown bag it" to work, or anywhere else, you'll find these fillings offer a good variety. They are easy to make and will keep several days under refrigeration. Be sure to use the quantity stated because the calories add up fast. Always use thin-sliced rye, whole wheat, or white bread that has no more than 40 calories per slice. See if you can leave one slice behind and eat the sandwich open-faced. If not, at least that extra slice is only 40 calories, which has been calculated into the daily calorie count.

Cucumber Filling
    3 ounces cream cheese
    1 teaspoon cold water
    2 cucumbers, grated
    ¼ cup minced green onion tops
    1 drop green food coloring

Whip the cream cheese until fluffy. Put in a mixing bowl and blend in the remaining ingredients. Chill.
Makes filling for 4 sandwiches.

CALORIES: 93.3   CALCIUM: 29.5 mg.
PROTEIN: 2.2 gm.   SODIUM: 61 mg.
CARBOHYDRATE: 3.6 gm.   CHOLESTEROL: 27 mg.
FAT: 8 gm.

Watercress Sandwich Filling

    ½ cup finely chopped watercress, stems removed
    3 tablespoons diet mayonnaise
    Dash paprika

Blend the ingredients.
Makes filling for 2 sandwiches.

CALORIES: 39
PROTEIN: .8 gm.
CARBOHYDRATE: 2.1 gm.
FAT: 3.1 gm.

CALCIUM: 40 mg.
SODIUM: 41 mg.
CHOLESTEROL: 0 mg.

Onion Sandwich Filling

    1½ cups cottage cheese
    3 tablespoons yogurt
    3 tablespoons minced parsley
    ¼ cup minced green onions, tops and bottoms

Put the cottage cheese in a food processor with the yogurt. Blend until smooth. Remove and put in a mixing bowl. Blend in the onions and parsley. Chill.
Makes filling for 4 sandwiches.

CALORIES: 55.4
PROTEIN: 13 gm.
CARBOHYDRATE: 2.9 gm.
FAT: 4 gm.

CALCIUM: 53 mg.
SODIUM: 188 mg.
CHOLESTEROL: 8 mg.

Danish Sea Sandwich Filling

    3 ounces cream cheese, whipped
    1 tablespoon yogurt
    1 cup pickled herring tidbits
    1 small onion, minced
    1 packet lo-cal sweetener
    ¼ teaspoon white pepper
    1 tablespoon vinegar
    1 apple, chopped fine
    Dark rye or pumpernickel bread

Place the ingredients in a mixing bowl and gently mix. Chill. Put on dark rye or pumpernickel bread.
Makes filling for 6 sandwiches.

CALORIES: 88.3   CALCIUM: 12.8 mg.
PROTEIN: 1.4 gm.   SODIUM: 37.5 mg.
CARBOHYDRATE: 3.7 gm.   CHOLESTEROL: 46.1 mg.
FAT: 6.7 gm.

Shrimp Salad Sandwich Filling
 1 cup cooked small shrimp
 1/2 cup chopped cooked asparagus
 1/2 cup diet mayonnaise
 Pepper

Mix the first three ingredients and season to taste with pepper.
Makes filling for 4 sandwiches.

CALORIES: 63.4   CALCIUM: 43.5 mg.
PROTEIN: 8.4 gm.   SODIUM: 38 mg.
CARBOHYDRATE: 1.9 gm.   CHOLESTEROL: 90 mg.
FAT: 2.3 gm.

Crab Sandwich Filling
 1 cup cooked crabmeat
 3 tablespoons minced green onion tops
 1/4 cup diet mayonnaise
 1 tablespoon plain yogurt
 1/2 teaspoon seafood seasoning
 1 hard-cooked egg, chopped
 Pumpernickel bread

Mix all the ingredients and put open-faced on pumpernickel bread.
Makes filling for 4 sandwiches.

CALORIES: 62   CALCIUM: 24 mg.
PROTEIN: 6.9 gm.   SODIUM: 36.2 mg.
CARBOHYDRATE: 1.3 gm. CHOLESTEROL: 153.5 mg.
FAT: 3.2 gm.

Smoked Oyster Sandwich Filling

    1 3-ounce can smoked oysters
    3 ounces whipped cream cheese
    1 tablespoon minced onion
    2 strips bacon, crumbled

Mix all the ingredients.
Makes filling for 4 sandwiches.

CALORIES: 94   CALCIUM: 33.8 mg.
PROTEIN: 3.5 gm.   SODIUM: 79 mg.
CARBOHYDRATE: 1.3 gm.   CHOLESTEROL: 63.2 mg.
FAT: 8.4 gm.

Chicken Curry Sandwich Filling

    1 cup cooked chicken
    1/4 cup diet mayonnaise
    1 tablespoon plain yogurt
    2 teaspoons curry
    3 tablespoons chopped green onion
    1 hard-cooked egg, chopped

Mix all the ingredients in a mixing bowl.
Makes filling for 4 sandwiches.

CALORIES: 91.2   CALCIUM: 14.5 mg.
PROTEIN: 13 gm.   SODIUM: 59 mg.
CARBOHYDRATE: 1 gm.   CHOLESTEROL: 109.2 mg.
FAT: 4.3 gm.

Cobb Salad Sandwich Filling

    1 avocado, diced
    1 stalk rib celery, sliced thin
    1 hard-cooked egg, chopped fine
    1/2 cup fresh bean sprouts, chopped
    1/4 cup chopped tomato
    1/4 cup chopped green onion
    Dash white pepper
    Dash garlic powder

2 tablespoons diet Thousand Island dressing
4 lettuce leaves
4 slices thin rye bread
Dash paprika

Mix all the ingredients in a bowl. To serve, put a lettuce leaf on each of the 4 pieces of bread and divide the mixture into 4 portions. Spread on the bread. Garnish with a sprinkle of paprika and serve open-faced.
Serves 4.

CALORIES: 175   CALCIUM: 12 mg.
PROTEIN: 7 gm.   SODIUM: 18 mg.
CARBOHYDRATE: 4 gm.   CHOLESTEROL: 65 mg.
FAT: 10 gm.

Egg White Sandwich Filling

4 cooked egg whites, chopped
2 tablespoons diet Thousand Island dressing
1 tablespoon minced green onion
Thin-sliced bread

Put all the ingredients in a small bowl and mix well. Serve on thin-sliced bread.
Serves 4.

CALORIES: 32   CALCIUM: 3 mg.
PROTEIN: 4 gm.   SODIUM: 48 mg.
CARBOHYDRATE: .3 gm.   CHOLESTEROL: 0 mg.
FAT: Trace gm.

12

Fruits

At the Naval Academy, fruit became the favorite of the midshipmen. They often remarked that they used to carry a bag of potato chips in their briefcases for a snack but that they had switched to apples and oranges. That was music to my ears.

The fruit I served the most was, of course, melon. The melon is low in calories and high in taste and texture. A whole cantaloupe that is 5 inches in diameter contains 159 calories; a casaba melon 6½ inches in diameter contains 367 calories—remember, this is for the whole fruit. That's a lot of quantity for the number of calories. Nearly all the recipes that follow use this wonderful fruit.

Broiled Coconut Casaba

    1 casaba melon
    1 orange
    1 tangerine
    2 tablespoons diet peach jam
    1 tablespoon water
    ½ cup shredded coconut

Cut the melon into 8 slices. Cut 4 of the slices into chunks. Cut the remaining 4 slices in half. Peel the orange and tangerine and cut into sections. Cut each of these sections in half. Mix the oranges,

tangerines, and cut-up casaba melon in a bowl. Place the casaba slices in a baking dish and top with the fruit. Meanwhile, heat the peach jam and water and brush on the fruit. Top with coconut and put under broiler for 2 minutes.
Serves 8.

CALORIES: 81.2
PROTEIN: 2.5 gm.
CARBOHYDRATE: 14.8 gm.
FAT: 1.8 gm.

CALCIUM: 35.5 mg.
SODIUM: 11 mg.
CHOLESTEROL: 0 mg.

Broiled Grapefruit with Melon
2 pink grapefruit
½ cup cantaloupe puree

Cut the grapefruit in half and loosen the meat from the peel with a grapefruit knife. Spread the cantaloupe puree over each half. Put under broiler for 5 minutes. Serve hot.
Serves 4.

CALORIES: 68.2
PROTEIN: .4 gm.
CARBOHYDRATE: 6.3 gm.
FAT: .05 gm.

CALCIUM: 10.5 mg.
SODIUM: 6 mg.
CHOLESTEROL: 0 mg.

Broiled Melon
2 small cantaloupes
2 teaspoons honey
1 tablespoon water

Cut the cantaloupes in half and scoop out the seeds. Heat the honey and water and brush on the cantaloupe. Put under the broiler for 5 minutes.
Serves 4.

CALORIES: 92
PROTEIN: .3 gm.
CARBOHYDRATE: 23.1 gm.
FAT: .3 gm.

CALCIUM: 38.7 mg.
SODIUM: 19 mg.
CHOLESTEROL: 0 mg.

Karen's Oranges in Melon Cups

    4 large oranges, sliced
    2 tablespoons honey
    1 cantaloupe, cut into quarters
    Fresh mint sprigs

Peel the oranges so that none of the white membrane is left on them. Slice. Layer the slices in a bowl and pour the honey over them. Chill 2 hours. Turn the slices in the honey and the juice that will have leached from the oranges. Chill another hour. Serve over quarters of cantaloupe that have been cleaned and peeled. Garnish with sprigs of fresh mint.
Serves 4.

CALORIES: 128
PROTEIN: 2.35 gm.
CARBOHYDRATE: 8.2 gm.
FAT: .3 gm.

CALCIUM: 78 mg.
SODIUM: 25 mg.
CHOLESTEROL: 0 mg.

Apple Melon Bake

    4 apples
    1 cantaloupe
    2 tablespoons diet margarine
    4 packets lo-cal sweetener
    2 teaspoons cinnamon
    1/3 cup orange juice

Peel and core the apples and cut them in half. Peel the cantaloupe and cut into thick slices. Place the apple and cantaloupe slices in a glass baking dish. In a small saucepan, melt the diet margarine. Stir in the lo-cal sweetener, cinnamon, and orange juice. Pour over the fruit. Bake uncovered for 25 minutes in an oven set at 300 degrees. Serve hot.
Serves 4.

CALORIES: 158.1
PROTEIN: 1.3 gm.
CARBOHYDRATE: 27.7 gm.
FAT: 3.8 gm.

CALCIUM: 29.9 mg.
SODIUM: 15 mg.
CHOLESTEROL: 0 mg.

Baked Pears in Melon

⅛ teaspoon cinnamon
Dash mace
1 tablespoon flour
2 packets lo-cal sweetener
1 tablespoon diet margarine
1 tablespoon lemon juice
8 slices cantaloupe
3 cups sliced pears

Mix the spices, sweetener, and flour together. Melt the diet margarine, add the lemon juice, and stir into the flour mixture. Put the cantaloupe slices in the bottom of a glass baking dish and top with the sliced pears. Pour the flour mixture over all and bake for 15 minutes in an oven set at 350 degrees.
Serves 6.

CALORIES: 67.5   CALCIUM: 12.7 mg.
PROTEIN: .7 gm.   SODIUM: 7 mg.
CARBOHYDRATE: 14.8 gm. CHOLESTEROL: 0 mg.
FAT: 1.3 gm.

Melon Coconut Kabob

1 cup cantaloupe, cut into chunks
1 cup watermelon, cut into chunks
½ cup honeydew, cut into chunks
2 tablespoons orange juice
½ cup shredded coconut

Put alternating colors of melon pieces onto wooden skewers. Sprinkle with orange juice and roll in coconut. Chill.
Serves 8.

CALORIES: 44.6   CALCIUM: 7.4 mg.
PROTEIN: .6 gm.   SODIUM: 4.8 mg.
CARBOHYDRATE: 4.8 gm.   CHOLESTEROL: 0 mg.
FAT: 28.6 gm.

Melon Cup

    2 small cantaloupes
    1 pint fresh raspberries
    ¼ teaspoon castor sugar
    Dash cinnamon
    Lemon leaves

Peel the cantaloupes and cut in half. Remove seeds and pat dry. Put
the raspberries in a bowl and sprinkle with sugar and cinnamon.
Stir. Fill the cantaloupe bowls with the raspberries. Garnish with
lemon leaves.
Serves 4.

CALORIES: 48
PROTEIN: 1.1 gm.
CARBOHYDRATE: 12 gm.
FAT: .2 gm.

CALCIUM: 22 mg.
SODIUM: 20 mg.
CHOLESTEROL: 0 mg.

Peach Melon Cup

    2 small cantaloupes
    3 cups peach slices
    ¼ teaspoon nutmeg
    Dash cinnamon
    Lemon leaves

Peel the cantaloupes and cut in half. Remove seeds and pat dry. Put
the peach slices in a bowl and sprinkle with the spices. Stir. Fill the
cantaloupe bowls with the peaches. Garnish with lemon leaves.
Serves 4.

CALORIES: 99
PROTEIN: 1.7 gm.
CARBOHYDRATE: 32.1 gm.
FAT: 1.5 gm.

CALCIUM: 49.2 mg.
SODIUM: 1.1 mg.
CHOLESTEROL: 1 mg.

Spiced Melon Plums

    1 large can plums
    Water
    1 piece stick cinnamon
    3 whole cloves
    1 whole allspice
    1/4 cup rosé wine
    2 teaspoons lemon juice
    1 cup melon balls

If the plums have been packed in a sugar syrup, rinse several times with water. If they are dietetic, save juice. Place plums in a large saucepan and add 1 can of water (or juice from dietetic plums). Add all remaining ingredients except the melon balls to the saucepan and bring to a boil. Turn down the heat and simmer 5 minutes. Remove from heat. Strain the juice. Place the plums in a serving bowl with the melon balls and pour the juice over the fruit. Chill. Serve hot or cold.
Serves 4.

CALORIES: 76.6
PROTEIN: .8 gm.
CARBOHYDRATE: 16.9 gm.
FAT: .4 gm.

CALCIUM: 17.4 mg.
SODIUM: 8 mg.
CHOLESTEROL: 0 mg.

Strawberries and Melon Balls

    2 cups sliced strawberries
    2 cups melon balls
    1/2 cup lychee nuts
    1/4 cup tangerine juice

Mix the fruits together in a bowl and pour tangerine juice over all.
Serves 6.

CALORIES: 41.7
PROTEIN: .8 gm.
CARBOHYDRATE: 9.9 gm.
FAT: .4 gm.

CALCIUM: 17.5 mg.
SODIUM: 7 mg.
CHOLESTEROL: 0 mg.

Orange Soufflé

1 recipe Soufflé Base
2 teaspoons orange flavor extract
2 teaspoons grated orange peel
3 tablespoons orange juice

Prepare 1 recipe Soufflé Base according to the directions on page 164. Add the remaining ingredients to the egg yolk mixture. Fold in the egg whites and place in a soufflé dish. Chill.
Serves 6.

CALORIES: 94.5
PROTEIN: 9.6 gm.
CARBOHYDRATE: 3.9 gm.
FAT: 3.7 gm.

CALCIUM: 58.8 mg.
SODIUM: 136 mg.
CHOLESTEROL: 46.1 mg.

Tangerine Melon Boat

2 small cantaloupes
1 tablespoon orange juice
1 tablespoon diet strawberry jam
3 tangerines
1/2 cup sliced peaches
1/2 cup kadota figs
1/2 cup fresh raspberries

Cut the cantaloupes into halves and clean and seed them. Pat dry. Mix the orange juice and the strawberry jam in a small bowl. Meanwhile, peel the tangerines and break into sections. Cut these sections into pieces and place in a mixing bowl. Combine the other fruit with the tangerines. Pour the jam mixture over all. Fill the cantaloupes with the fruit.
Serves 6.

CALORIES: 95.8
PROTEIN: .7 gm.
CARBOHYDRATE: 8.8 gm.
FAT: .3 gm.

CALCIUM: 19 mg.
SODIUM: 14 mg.
CHOLESTEROL: 0 mg.

13

Eggs

Eggs can be used in every course of a meal, from the appetizer to the dessert. In this book we have calculated the egg to contain 73 calories. Most of those calories are found at the center of the egg in the yolk. The egg white has only 15 calories and can be used in many ways when hard-cooked. For instance, it can be chopped and mixed with diet dressings or diet mayonnaise and then stuffed into cucumbers, celery, or zucchini. It is quick and easy to make and keep in the refrigerator for several days to use later.

Here are some important tips for cooking eggs. Never add milk or cream to scrambled eggs or omelets; it only makes the eggs tough. When you "fry" an egg for breakfast, spray your pan with vegetable spray and put the pan over medium heat. When the pan is heated put in the egg and let it cook until the white is slightly set and then add 1 tablespoon of water. Put the lid on the pan and wait for several seconds. The egg will be perfectly done. There is no need to turn the egg; just remove it from the pan.

Everyone knows how temperamental those nasty little white morsels can be. They crack when they shouldn't and break when you want them whole. You will get better results if you work with them at room temperature. If you are beating an egg white, it will triple in volume if it's beaten at room temperature in a copper bowl. Use a balloon whisk to beat eggs. You will find this implement a must in your kitchen.

Here is a pointer you should store away for frequent use: Never boil an egg. Does this statement shock you? There is a good reason for it: An egg that has been boiled is often improperly cooked. You peel off the shell, cut open the hard-cooked egg, and what do you see? An egg white and a yolk that has a thick green layer around it. This layer has not only an unappealing appearance but a nasty taste. So from now on put the eggs that are at room temperature into boiling water, bring the water back to a boil, cover the pan, and remove from the heat. Allow to set until the water is cold. Voilà! The perfect hard-cooked egg with *NO* green ring.

Egg Muffin with Canadian Bacon

1 slice Canadian bacon
1 egg
1 English muffin
1 ounce Velveeta cheese

In a skillet, sauté the Canadian bacon. Fry the egg, breaking the yolk. Cook until the egg is hard. Open the English muffin and place under the broiler. Top with Velveeta cheese. When cheese is melted, remove from broiler and top with Canadian bacon and egg. Serve as a sandwich.
Serves 1.

CALORIES: 313 CALCIUM: 169 mg.
PROTEIN: 20.3 gm. SODIUM: 1,096 mg.
CARBOHYDRATE: 12.4 gm. CHOLESTEROL: 342 mg.
FAT: 12 gm.

French Omelet

2 eggs
1 teaspoon water
Dash pepper
Dash salt substitute
Vegetable cooking spray

In a mixing bowl, beat the eggs slightly with the water. Add the pepper and salt substitute. Heat an omelet pan over high heat. Spray with vegetable cooking spray. From 10 inches above the pan slowly pour in the egg mixture. Count to 8, allowing the egg to set. Then shake and tilt the pan to allow the uncooked portion to go to the sides while pulling the cooked egg portion toward the center. When the egg is set, fold in half and turn onto a serving platter. *Serves 1.*

CALORIES: 146
PROTEIN: 12.4 gm.
CARBOHYDRATE: 18 gm.
FAT: 11 gm.

CALCIUM: 52 mg.
SODIUM: 132 mg.
CHOLESTEROL: 506 mg.

Fried Egg

Vegetable cooking spray
1 large whole egg
1 tablespoon water
Dash pepper

Lightly spray the bottom and sides of an 8-inch skillet with the vegetable cooking spray. Do not use any fats like butter, margarine, or lard. Heat the pan over medium heat. Break open the egg and cook 1 minute. Put 1 tablespoon of water into the pan and cover with a tight-fitting lid. Cook an additional 2 minutes or until the egg is cooked. Add a dash of pepper before serving. *Makes 1 egg.*

CALORIES: 73
PROTEIN: 6.2 gm.
CARBOHYDRATE: .4 gm.
FAT: 5.5 gm.

CALCIUM: 26 mg.
SODIUM: 61 mg.
CHOLESTEROL: 253 mg.

Mexican Puff

8 eggs
2 tablespoons flour
1 cup 2 percent milk
2 tablespoons sliced green onion tops
2 ounces green chilies
2 ounces Cheddar cheese, grated
Dash white pepper

In a mixing bowl beat the eggs, flour, and milk. Stir in the green onion tops, green chilies, and cheese. Add the white pepper. Pour into a 9-inch pie pan. Bake for 35 minutes or until puffed and set in an oven set at 350 degrees.
Serves 8.

CALORIES: 120
PROTEIN: 9.1 gm.
CARBOHYDRATE: 7.1 gm.
FAT: 5.7 gm.

CALCIUM: 135 mg.
SODIUM: 129.3 mg.
CHOLESTEROL: 266 mg.

Cheese Omelet

2 large whole eggs
1/2 teaspoon water
Dash pepper
Vegetable cooking spray
1 ounce Cheddar cheese, grated
2 teaspoons parsley flakes

In a small mixing bowl, beat the eggs slightly. Add the water and pepper and beat the egg mixture until it is frothy. Spray an 8-inch omelet pan with vegetable cooking spray. From about 10 inches above the pan slowly pour in the egg mixture. Count to 8 and, using a fork, stir the eggs as you would for scrambled eggs. Allow the egg mixture to sit for a moment and then use a spatula to pull the eggs into the center. Meanwhile, tilt the pan so that the uncooked portion of the eggs moves to the outer edges. Place the grated cheese and parsley flakes on one half of the egg mixture and carefully fold in half. Turn out onto a serving plate.
Serves 2.

CALORIES: 131
PROTEIN: 13.5 gm.
CARBOHYDRATE: 19.5 gm.
FAT: 10.6 gm.

CALCIUM: 210 mg.
SODIUM: 80 mg.
CHOLESTEROL: 264 mg.

Soft-Boiled Eggs
2 eggs

Place eggs in a saucepan and add enough water to generously cover the eggs. Turn the heat on medium and bring the water to a boil. Turn the heat down to simmer and wait 3 minutes. Serve the eggs in an egg cup. Cut off the top half and scoop out the egg. *Serves 2.*

CALORIES: 73
PROTEIN: 6.2 gm.
CARBOHYDRATE: .4 gm.
FAT: 5.5 gm.

CALCIUM: 26 mg.
SODIUM: 61 mg.
CHOLESTEROL: 253 mg.

Piperade
1 green pepper, thinly sliced
1 tomato, cut in wedges
1 clove garlic, minced
1 tablespoon minced parsley
Dash red pepper
1 teaspoon diet margarine
4 eggs, beaten
1 tablespoon 2 percent milk
2 slices thin diet bread, toasted

Sauté the green pepper, tomato, garlic, parsley, and red pepper in the diet margarine over low heat for 15 minutes until the vegetables are well cooked. Meanwhile, beat the eggs with the milk and scramble in a skillet. To serve, cut the toast into diamonds, place the eggs in the center of the serving plate, and surround them with the vegetable mixture. *Serves 4.*

CALORIES: 94
PROTEIN: 7.1 gm.
CARBOHYDRATE: 3.8 gm.
FAT: 5.6 gm.

CALCIUM: 42.2 mg.
SODIUM: 67.3 mg.
CHOLESTEROL: 253 mg.

14

Casseroles

$\mathbf{A}$s a rule, casseroles are a no-no. When eating out you must avoid ordering them at all costs. So many ingredients could have been added when making the sauce or some unknown food preparation technique used when preparing the main ingredient that you cannot be sure what you are getting. The waiter in most cases is unqualified to tell you just what went into the casserole. Also, many restaurants will use a frozen product and just heat it up, though they don't want to admit that it wasn't made fresh by their chef. It is just too risky to order it, given the extra calories you could be getting. When making the casseroles in this chapter, at least you will know the exact number of calories in each.

Beef Tacos

  1 pound ground beef
  1 teaspoon Worcestershire sauce
  1 onion, chopped
  1 tablespoon parsley, minced
  1 tablespoon chili powder
  ½ teaspoon paprika
  3 cloves garlic, minced
  ¼ cup tomato juice
  12 corn tortillas
  1½ cups shredded lettuce

1 onion, diced
1 tomato, chopped
1 1/2 cups Cheddar cheese, grated
12 teaspoons hot sauce

Place the ground beef, Worcestershire sauce, chopped onion, parsley, chili powder, paprika, and garlic in a skillet and sauté until the meat is done and the spices well blended. Stir in the tomato juice and simmer until the liquid is reduced. Keep warm. Meanwhile, steam the tortillas and keep them warm. To serve, put 2 tablespoons meat mixture into each steamed tortilla and garnish with 1/8 cup lettuce, 1 tablespoon diced onion, 1 tablespoon tomato, and 2 tablespoons Cheddar cheese. Roll up and serve with 1 teaspoon hot sauce.

Serves 6 persons 2 tacos each.

CALORIES: 228
PROTEIN: 19.3 gm.
CARBOHYDRATE: 13.3 gm.
FAT: 9.7 gm.

CALCIUM: 387.4 mg.
SODIUM: 645 mg.
CHOLESTEROL: 122 mg.

Quiche Lorraine

Vegetable cooking spray
4 ounces Swiss cheese, grated
1/4 cup chopped green onions
3 ounces Canadian bacon, chopped
3 eggs, beaten
1 1/2 cups 2 percent milk
2 tablespoons flour
1/8 teaspoon seafood seasoning

Spray a quiche dish with vegetable cooking spray. Spread the Swiss cheese over the bottom of the dish. Sprinkle the green onions and Canadian bacon over the cheese. In a mixing bowl, beat the eggs, milk, flour, and seafood seasoning until they are well blended. Pour over the cheese in the dish and place in an oven set at 350 degrees. Bake uncovered for 45 minutes until the custard is set.

Serves 6.

CALORIES: 164
PROTEIN: 13.55 gm.
CARBOHYDRATE: 9.86 gm.
FAT: 9.95 gm.

CALCIUM: 266 mg.
SODIUM: 471 mg.
CHOLESTEROL: 174 mg.

Welsh Rarebit

1 cup shredded American cheese
1 cup shredded Cheddar cheese
1 teaspoon Worcestershire sauce
1 teaspoon dry mustard
3 ounces lite beer
½ cup 2 percent milk
6 slices diet white bread

In a saucepan, melt the cheese with the Worcestershire sauce, mustard, and beer. When melted and well blended pour in the milk. Blend and keep mixture warm. Meanwhile, toast the bread in the oven until well browned. To serve, cut bread into triangles and serve 2 triangles (1 slice bread) per person. Pour cheese mixture over triangles.
Serves 6.

CALORIES: 207
PROTEIN: 11.7 gm.
CARBOHYDRATE: 12.3 gm.
FAT: 12.7 gm.

CALCIUM: 303 mg.
SODIUM: 385 mg.
CHOLESTEROL: 61 mg.

15

Vegetables

You cannot imagine the midshipmen's dislike for vegetables. I thought it amusing that they considered vegetables a necessary evil in nutrition. Sometimes they would pick at and play with the vegetables. One football player actually spent at least fifteen minutes separating the onions, green peppers, and tomatoes from one of the recipes. He was disgusted that I had put them all together in a recipe and then had the nerve to tell him that he had to eat it. Though he went hungry that meal, he still asked me if other dishes would contain these foreign critters. Some of the young mids even went so far as to tell me that they were allergic to vegetables. But once we got into the diet, the midshipmen changed their minds. I added spices and melon balls and more spices in an effort to win them over to vegetables. After several days I heard no more complaints.

If you would like to add another vegetable to the menu, remember that you can't add yams, sweet corn, or sweet peas. These vegetables contain a great amount of natural sugar, and we are trying to cut down on sugar. But trading one plain vegetable for another is fine. Cooked celery or braised cucumbers are good substitutions. Brussels sprouts, cauliflower, turnips, and beets are palate-pleasing vegetables that are often overlooked. You may say "Ugh!" but I say "Think thin."

Any of the plain vegetables are delicious raw. They are great for lunches and late-night snacks.

If you decide at mealtime that you have to have a larger portion of food, make that larger portion a vegetable (or salad) and I promise that you won't turn into a rabbit!

Acorn Squash

    1 acorn squash
    1 teaspoon basil
    2 teaspoons diet margarine
    Pepper

Cut the acorn squash in half. Spread each half with diet margarine. Sprinkle with basil and pepper. Place in a baking dish and cover with foil. Place in an oven set at 350 degrees. Bake for 60 minutes or until the squash is tender.
Serves 4.

CALORIES: 115.5   CALCIUM: 44 mg.
PROTEIN: 2.3 gm.   SODIUM: 1 mg.
CARBOHYDRATE: 25 gm. CHOLESTEROL: 0 mg.
FAT: .6 gm.

Asparagus Tips

    1 pound asparagus
    1 tablespoon diet margarine
    ¼ cup beef bouillon
    ¼ teaspoon pepper

Clean and trim the asparagus and peel stems up to the flower. Melt the diet margarine in a saucepan and sauté the asparagus for 3 minutes. Pour in the beef bouillon and pepper. Bring the bouillon to a boil and cover the pan. Turn down the heat and simmer for 12 minutes or until the asparagus is tender.
Serves 4.

CALORIES: 42   CALCIUM: 25 mg.
PROTEIN: 2.8 gm.   SODIUM: 62 mg.
CARBOHYDRATE: 5.7 gm. CHOLESTEROL: 0 mg.
FAT: 3.4 gm.

Baked Fennel

2 large fennel
1 tablespoon diet margarine
⅛ teaspoon pepper
¼ teaspoon oregano leaves

Prepare the fennel by cutting off the long tops and slicing the base from the bottom of the fennel bulb. Discard any darkened leaves. Wash in cold water and cut into quarters. Place the fennel in a saucepan and cover with water. Cook over medium-high heat 12 minutes until slightly tender. Drain and pat dry. Place in a baking dish and dot with the diet margarine. Sprinkle with the pepper and oregano. Cover and bake 15 minutes in an oven set at 350 degrees. *Serves 4.*

CALORIES: 40.5
PROTEIN: 2.3 gm.
CARBOHYDRATE: 3.9 gm.
FAT: .5 gm.

CALCIUM: 25 mg.
SODIUM: 4 mg.
CHOLESTEROL: 0 mg.

Baked Tomatoes Parmesan

4 tomatoes, cut in half
2 tablespoons cracker crumbs
4 tablespoons Parmesan cheese
2 teaspoons dry parsley
Pepper

Place the tomato halves in a baking dish and sprinkle with the cracker crumbs, Parmesan cheese, parsley, and pepper. Bake for 25 minutes or until the tomatoes are done in an oven set at 350 degrees. *Serves 4.*

CALORIES: 51.9
PROTEIN: 6.79 gm.
CARBOHYDRATE: 8.8 gm.
FAT: 4.15 gm.

CALCIUM: 180.4 mg.
SODIUM: 75 mg.
CHOLESTEROL: 11 mg.

Broccoli Sauté

1 pound fresh broccoli
1 tablespoon diet margarine, melted
Dash ground red pepper

Clean the broccoli and cut up. Remove the tough ends and leaves. Use a potato peeler to peel the broccoli up to the flowers. Place the broccoli in a small skillet with the margarine. Sprinkle with the red pepper. Sauté 12 minutes in the skillet over medium-high heat or until the broccoli is done but still crisp.
Serves 4.

CALORIES: 38.5
PROTEIN: 4 gm.
CARBOHYDRATE: 6.7 gm.
FAT: 1.3 gm.

CALCIUM: 116.7 mg.
SODIUM: 17 mg.
CHOLESTEROL: 0 mg.

Brussels Sprouts

1 pound Brussels sprouts
½ teaspoon white pepper
¼ cup water
1 teaspoon lemon juice
1 tablespoon diet margarine
1 teaspoon basil

Place all the ingredients in a saucepan, cover, and bring the water to a boil. Cook 10 minutes over medium heat until the vegetables are tender.
Serves 6.

CALORIES: 49.1
PROTEIN: 4.7 gm.
CARBOHYDRATE: 7.3 gm.
FAT: 1.5 gm.

CALCIUM: 36.2 mg.
SODIUM: 16 mg.
CHOLESTEROL: 0 mg.

Sautéed Cucumbers

    3 tablespoons diet margarine
    ½ teaspoon white wine vinegar
    ½ teaspoon basil
    ½ teaspoon white pepper
    3 tablespoons beef bouillon
    5 cups sliced cucumbers
    2 tablespoons minced parsley

In a saucepan melt the diet margarine. Stir in the wine vinegar, basil, white pepper, and beef bouillon. When hot, add the cucumbers. Over high heat and stirring and tossing constantly cook the cucumbers for 8 minutes. Sprinkle with parsley.
Serves 4.

CALORIES: 36　　　　　　CALCIUM: 32.5 mg.
PROTEIN: 2 gm.　　　　　SODIUM: 31 mg.
CARBOHYDRATE: 1.2 gm.　CHOLESTEROL: 0 mg.
FAT: 5 gm.

Carrots Vichy

    2 cups peeled and sliced carrots
    2 cups water
    Dash white pepper
    1 packet lo-cal sweetener
    ¼ teaspoon dried dill

In a small saucepan place the peeled and sliced carrots. Add the water, pepper, and lo-cal sweetener. Bring the water to a boil and boil uncovered until the water is nearly gone. The carrots should be tender. If they are still not tender enough, add ½ cup more water and continue to cook until done. Before serving, sprinkle with dill.
Makes 4 ½-cup servings.

CALORIES: 11.8　　　　　CALCIUM: 37 mg.
PROTEIN: 1.1 gm.　　　　SODIUM: 22 mg.
CARBOHYDRATE: 9.7 gm.　CHOLESTEROL: 0 mg.
FAT: 2 gm.

Crookneck Squash

    4 crookneck squash
    1/2 cup water
    2 tablespoons chopped chives
    Pepper
    1/4 teaspoon thyme
    Dash garlic powder

Slice the crookneck squash and place in a saucepan. Add 1/2 cup water and the chopped chives. Sprinkle with pepper and the remaining herbs. Cover. Bring the water to a boil and then turn down the heat to simmer. Cook 12 minutes or until the squash are done. *Serves 4.*

CALORIES: 7.5
PROTEIN: .45 gm.
CARBOHYDRATE: .23 gm.
FAT: Trace

CALCIUM: 1.4 mg.
SODIUM: 1 mg.
CHOLESTEROL: 0 mg.

Red Cabbage

    1/4 cup chicken bouillon
    1/4 cup water
    1/4 cup sliced green onions
    3 tablespoons red wine vinegar
    1/4 cup applesauce
    1/4 teaspoon ground cloves
    2 cups shredded red cabbage

Put all ingredients but the cabbage in a medium saucepan. Bring to a boil and add the red cabbage. Stir well. Return to a boil and then reduce the heat to low. Cover and simmer 40 minutes until the liquid has evaporated.
Serves 4.

CALORIES: 23.1
PROTEIN: 1 gm.
CARBOHYDRATE: 4.7 gm.
FAT: .3 gm.

CALCIUM: 17.6 mg.
SODIUM: 67 mg.
CHOLESTEROL: 0 mg.

Spaghetti Squash

1 spaghetti squash
½ teaspoon paprika
⅛ teaspoon pepper
Pinch garlic powder

Fill a large saucepan with water and add the spaghetti squash, paprika, pepper, and garlic powder. Bring the water to a boil and cover. Turn down the heat and simmer for 1 hour or until squash is done. Remove from the water and cut in half. Using a fork pull the squash in strings from the center of the squash. It will look like spaghetti.
Serves 4.

CALORIES: 14.5   CALCIUM: 22.5 mg.
PROTEIN: .6 gm.   SODIUM: 1 mg.
CARBOHYDRATE: 3.4 gm.   CHOLESTEROL: 0 mg.
FAT: .1 gm.

Zucchini and Tomatoes

1 tablespoon diet margarine
⅓ cup chopped onion
¼ cup parsley, no stems
2 cloves garlic, pressed
2 cups sliced zucchini
1 medium tomato, diced
¼ teaspoon salt
⅛ teaspoon pepper

In a medium saucepan, melt the diet margarine. Add the onion and sauté until clear. Meanwhile, whirl the parsley and garlic in a food processor fitted with a steel blade. Add the parsley-garlic mixture, zucchini, and tomato to the onions and simmer over medium heat for 4 minutes. Add the salt and pepper. Cover and simmer an additional 12 minutes until the zucchini are done.
Serves 4.

CALORIES: 47.8   CALCIUM: 55 mg.
PROTEIN: 2.1 gm.   SODIUM: 138 mg.
CARBOHYDRATE: 7.53 gm.   CHOLESTEROL: 0 mg.
FAT: 1.65 gm.

16

Pasta, Potatoes, and Rice

When most people review the Annapolis Diet menu they are amazed to find recipes for pasta, potatoes, and rice. But you know the old saying, "Everything in moderation." A ½-cup serving of rice or pasta is not too many calories for anyone on a diet, and it really satisfies the desire for starch. A potato isn't fattening; it's what goes on it that makes for so many calories. There are some fine butter substitutes with hardly any calories that taste great. So our rule of thumb regarding pasta, potatoes, and rice is prepare it, eat it, and love it.

Here are a few of the midshipmen's favorites that won't add any inches to your hips.

Potatoes

Parmesan Potato Wedges
> 2 baking potatoes
> 2 tablespoons diet margarine
> 2 teaspoons chopped chives
> ¼ teaspoon white pepper
> 1½ ounces Parmesan cheese

Bake the potatoes in an oven set at 450 degrees 1 hour or until done. Remove from oven and cool. Cut into quarters. Melt the diet margarine and stir in the chives and pepper. Brush onto the potato wedges and then sprinkle wedges with the Parmesan cheese. Place the wedges in a baking pan and bake for 7 minutes or until the cheese has melted and the potatoes are lightly browned in an oven set at 500 degrees.
Serves 4.

CALORIES: 105   CALCIUM: 104.8 mg.
PROTEIN: 4.4 gm.   SODIUM: 96 mg.
CARBOHYDRATE: 10.6 gm.   CHOLESTEROL: 19 mg.
FAT: 2.3 gm.

Potatoes au Gratin

2 teaspoons diet margarine
1 small onion, sliced
1 tablespoon flour
¼ cup 2 percent milk
¼ teaspoon white pepper
2 ounces Velveeta cheese, grated
2 medium potatoes, baked

Melt the diet margarine in a small skillet. Sauté the onion until clear. Stir in the flour and milk. Add the white pepper and Velveeta cheese. Turn the heat down to low and cook until the cheese melts and the sauce is well blended. Slice the cooled baked potatoes and place in a small casserole. Pour the cheese sauce over the potatoes and cover. Bake for 25 minutes or until browned in an oven set at 350 degrees.
Serves 4.

CALORIES: 76   CALCIUM: 29.9 mg.
PROTEIN: 4 gm.   SODIUM: 166 mg.
CARBOHYDRATE: 14.8 gm.   CHOLESTEROL: 22.4 mg.
FAT: 1 gm.

Potato Skins

>   2 large baking potatoes
>   Black pepper
>   ¼ teaspoon oregano
>   2 tablespoons diet margarine

Bake the potatoes 1 hour or until done. Cut in half lengthwise. Scoop out the flesh and reserve for a later use, but leave a thin layer of flesh in the cavity. Sprinkle the inside of the cavity with pepper and oregano. Rub the outside of the skin with the diet margarine. Place on a baking sheet and return to the oven. Roast at 475 degrees for 20 minutes or until well browned and crisp.
Serves 4.

CALORIES: 33.3
PROTEIN: Trace
CARBOHYDRATE: Trace
FAT: 3.3 gm.

CALCIUM: Trace
SODIUM: 3 mg.
CHOLESTEROL: 0 mg.

Pasta

Fettuccine Karina

>   2 tablespoons diet margarine
>   1 clove garlic, minced
>   3 tablespoons parsley, minced
>   2 tablespoons chopped onion
>   White pepper
>   ½ cup 2 percent milk
>   2 cups cooked fettuccine

In a saucepan, melt the diet margarine. Add the garlic, parsley, onion, and white pepper. Sauté over medium-high heat for 4 minutes or until the vegetables are limp. Pour in the milk and bring to a boil. Toss with the fettuccine noodles and heat through.
Serves 4.

CALORIES: 132.6
PROTEIN: 4.6 gm.
CARBOHYDRATE: 20.3 gm.
FAT: 4 gm.

CALCIUM: 100 mg.
SODIUM: 21 mg.
CHOLESTEROL: 2 mg.

Hot Buttered Pasta

3 tablespoons diet margarine
1/2 teaspoon oregano
1 tablespoon dry parsley flakes
1/4 teaspoon white pepper
2 cups cooked spaghetti noodles

In a saucepan, melt the diet margarine. Add the seasonings and then toss with the noodles. Heat through.
Serves 4.

CALORIES: 115   CALCIUM: 10.5 mg.
PROTEIN: 2.4 gm.   SODIUM: 2 mg.
CARBOHYDRATE: 16.1 gm. CHOLESTEROL: 0 mg.
FAT: 4.8 gm.

Apricot Melon Noodles

1 quart water
8 ounces broad egg noodles
2 ounces cottage cheese
1/4 cup 2 percent milk
1/2 cup canned apricot halves
1 cup watermelon balls

Put the water in a saucepan and bring to a boil. Add the noodles and cook 15 minutes or until the noodles are just tender. Put the cottage cheese and milk in a food processor fitted with a steel blade and whirl until the mixture is pureed. Chop the apricot halves. Drain the cooked noodles and stir in the cheese puree. Fold in the chopped apricots and melon balls. Toss lightly and heat through.
Serves 4.

CALORIES: 96.2   CALCIUM: 46 mg.
PROTEIN: 4.6 gm.   SODIUM: 30 mg.
CARBOHYDRATE: 16.1 gm. CHOLESTEROL: 2 mg.
FAT: 1.6 gm.

Linguini in Clam Sauce

    1 tablespoon diet margarine
    1 1/2 tablespoons flour
    1/2 cup 2 percent milk
    1/2 cup water
    1/4 teaspoon white pepper
    1/3 teaspoon dry mustard
    1 1/2 cups cooked spaghetti noodles
    8 ounces cooked clams

In a saucepan, melt the diet margarine and then stir in the flour. Cook over medium heat for 4 minutes, stirring all the while. Using a whisk stir in the milk and water. Add the white pepper and dry mustard and cook the mixture over medium heat until the mixture is thickened. Stir in the cooked noodles and clams. Toss together and serve hot.
Serves 4.

CALORIES: 103
PROTEIN: 7.23 gm.
CARBOHYDRATE: 12.6 gm.
FAT: 4.1 gm.

CALCIUM: 71.25 mg.
SODIUM: 19 mg.
CHOLESTEROL: 92 mg.

Linguini and Melon in Clam Sauce

    8 ounces linguini
    2 tablespoons diet margarine
    1 tablespoon flour
    1 7-ounce can clams
    1/4 cup 2 percent milk
    1/2 cup cantaloupe balls
    1/4 cup Parmesan cheese
    1 tablespoon parsley, minced

Cook the linguini in boiling water until it is done. Drain. Meanwhile, in a saucepan melt the diet margarine and stir in the flour. Cook over medium heat for 3 minutes. Stir in the clams and the clam juice. Cook 5 minutes. Stir in the milk. Put the linguini on a

serving platter and top with the clam sauce. Top with the melon balls and sprinkle with Parmesan cheese and parsley.
Serves 4.

CALORIES: 103	CALCIUM: 71.2 mg.
PROTEIN: 7.2 gm.	SODIUM: 28 mg.
CARBOHYDRATE: 12.6 gm.	CHOLESTEROL: 80 mg.
FAT: 4.1 gm.	

Shells with Peas and Mushrooms

1 1/2 tablespoons diet margarine
1 tablespoon flour
1/4 teaspoon white pepper
1/2 teaspoon thyme
1/2 teaspoon oregano
1/4 teaspoon basil
1/4 teaspoon rosemary
2 cloves garlic, minced
1/2 cup 2 percent milk
1/4 cup white wine
10 ounces frozen peas
2 cups sliced mushrooms
2 cups cooked macaroni shells
Vegetable cooking spray
1 ounce Parmesan cheese, grated

In a saucepan, melt the margarine and stir in the flour. Cook this roux for 3 minutes and then stir in the seasonings and milk. Cook until the sauce is thickened and then add the wine, peas, and mushrooms. Heat through. Stir in the shells. Pour into a casserole dish that has been sprayed with vegetable cooking spray. Sprinkle with the grated Parmesan cheese and place uncovered in an oven set at 350 degree for 25 minutes. Serve hot.
Serves 4.

CALORIES: 231	CALCIUM: 149 mg.
PROTEIN: 36.6 gm.	SODIUM: 179 mg.
CARBOHYDRATE: 71.9 gm.	CHOLESTEROL: 13 mg.
FAT: 5.7 gm.	

Rice

Rice Pilaf

    1 tablespoon diet margarine
    3 tablespoons minced onion
    ¾ cup raw rice
    ¼ teaspoon pepper
    1½ cups chicken bouillon

Melt the diet margarine in a small pan. Add the onion and rice and cook until rice is brown. Add the pepper and pour in the chicken bouillon. Bring to a boil. Turn the heat down to low and cover. Simmer over low heat for 25 minutes.
Serves 6.

CALORIES: 124   CALCIUM: 9.5 mg.
PROTEIN: 5.5 gm.   SODIUM: 241 mg.
CARBOHYDRATE: 31.3 gm. CHOLESTEROL: 0 mg.
FAT: 3.5 gm.

Steamed Rice

    1 cup raw rice
    Water

Place the rice in a small saucepan. Add water until it covers the rice 1⅓ inches. Bring the water to a boil. Watch and listen carefully. When you can no longer hear the water boiling and the rice is picked with holes, remove the pan from the heat and cover. Set 15 minutes. Rice will be sticky, as in Oriental rice.
Serves 6.

CALORIES: 79   CALCIUM: 8 mg.
PROTEIN: 2.2 gm.   SODIUM: 2 mg.
CARBOHYDRATE: 26.3 gm. CHOLESTEROL: 0 mg.
FAT: .1 gm.

Saffron Rice

2 cups chicken broth
1/4 teaspoon saffron
2 teaspoons diet margarine
1/8 teaspoon white pepper
1 cup raw rice

In a saucepan, bring the chicken broth to a boil with the saffron, margarine, and white pepper. Stir in the raw rice and return to a boil. Turn down the heat to low. Cover the saucepan and cook for 25 minutes without removing the lid.
Serves 6.

CALORIES: 101
PROTEIN: 2.6 gm.
CARBOHYDRATE: 21.7 gm.
FAT: .6 gm.

CALCIUM: 24.8 mg.
SODIUM: 69 mg.
CHOLESTEROL: 13 mg.

Melon Brown Rice Pilaf

1 tablespoon diet margarine
1 cup rice
2 tablespoons chopped parsley
1/4 cup chopped onion
2 cups beef broth
1 cup melon balls

In a saucepan, melt the diet margarine and add the rice, parsley, and onion. Sauté the mixture for 6 minutes or until rice is lightly browned. Pour the beef broth over the rice mixture. Bring the mixture to a boil, turn down the heat, and cover. Simmer over low heat for 35 to 40 minutes or until the rice is done. Stir in the melon balls.
Makes 6 1/2-cup servings.

CALORIES: 154.7
PROTEIN: 2.7 gm.
CARBOHYDRATE: 29.5 gm.
FAT: 1.3 gm.

CALCIUM: 13.7 mg.
SODIUM: 267 mg.
CHOLESTEROL: 0 mg.

Risotto

    2 tablespoons diet margarine
    1 onion, chopped
    1/8 teaspoon white pepper
    1 1/2 cups rice, preferably short-grain white rice
    2 ounces dry white wine
    5 cups hot chicken broth
    1 1/2 cups water
    1 ounce Parmesan cheese, grated

In a saucepan, melt the diet margarine, add the onion and white pepper. Sauté over medium heat until clear. Add rice and stir to coat the rice with the butter-onion mixture. Pour in the wine and cook for 10 minutes, stirring constantly. Add 1 cup of the broth and 1/4 cup of the water. Cook until broth is absorbed, stirring frequently. Continue adding broth and water alternately until there is 1 cup of broth left. Add the last cup of broth to the cooked rice and stir in the Parmesan cheese. Heat through, cover, and allow to rest for 5 minutes.
Serves 6.

CALORIES: 125.2   CALCIUM: 34 mg.
PROTEIN: 4.2 gm.   SODIUM: 646 mg.
CARBOHYDRATE: 21.9 gm.   CHOLESTEROL: 8 mg.
FAT: 6 gm.

17

Fish and Shellfish

After a few weeks in the Naval Academy Diet Room, the mids started calling me "Chef Flipper." I loved it. It meant that they were having fun with the diet.

As a matter of fact, nearly all of the people on this diet began by telling me that their least favorite food was fish and that the only way they liked it was deep fried. At that moment I was the only one in the room who knew that they were about to have fish nearly every day for the next six weeks of their lives. I nearly panicked. For the first time the phrase "sink or swim" came quickly to mind. How could I tell them this news on the first day of their exciting new diet? Telling them that they would learn to love it many other ways than deep fried was my attempt at a diplomatic response.

I decided that I would give my "for the love of fish" talk. When dieting, it is important that your mouth be satisfied as well as your stomach. Actually, many of us could probably just taste the food and never swallow it and be totally satisfied. How many times have you said "Oh! If I could just have one bite of that." What you really wanted to do was taste that food, not fill your stomach with it. Right?

But fish is not only tasty. It's also especially low in calories. When lecturing on dieting, I love to compare the calories in 4 ounces of fish with the calories in 4 ounces of popular meats:

COMPARISON OF FISH TO MEAT
4-OUNCE SERVINGS

Fish	Calories	Meat	Calories
crab	105	top sirloin	243
tuna	120	leg of lamb	251
salmon	194	roast pork	276
cod fish	193	filet mignon	243
clams	33	hamburger	248

COMPARISON OF FISH TO FISH
4-OUNCE SERVINGS

Fish	Calories	Fish	Calories
tuna	120	oysters	86
trout	273	perch	134
bass	222	cod	193
sturgeon	169	sole	90
mackerel	268	haddock	80

It did not take the midshipmen long to discover that there were many fish entrées they liked. Each entrée was sufficiently seasoned to give it the extra zip it needed to satisfy the red meat eater. You will thus find the recipes in this chapter tasty as well as low-calorie.

Here are some important tips for preparing fish. First and most important, it must be fresh. Second, don't over-cook it. When you prepare shrimp or other shellfish, for instance, stop cooking it the minute it turns pink. If you wait too long, it turns tough as nails and the good flavor is gone. Use fresh lemon when cooking with fish. If you are poaching the fish, add some fresh celery leaves to the liquid. They will absorb the fish odor, leaving your kitchen and house smelling fresh.

Crab, shrimp, and lobster can be quite expensive, though they're really inexpensive when you prepare only 3 ounces at a time. You don't have to be a Rockefeller to afford 3 or 4 ounces, and the few calories in these items make them irresistible to dieters. But if you are on a low-cholesterol diet, be careful.

If you are dining out and you have a choice of red meat, poultry, or fish, always choose fish. You won't use up your daily calories in one bite and your stomach will be just as satisfied.

Cod Cohasset

4 4-ounce pieces cod, sole, or haddock
4 tablespoons diet mayonnaise
2 tablespoons parsley flakes
3 tablespoons cracker crumbs
1/4 teaspoon seafood seasoning
1/4 cup Parmesan cheese
2 tablespoons diet margarine
2 teaspoons lemon juice

Place cod in a baking dish. Spread 1 tablespoon diet margarine over each of the pieces. Sprinkle with parsley flakes, cracker crumbs, seafood seasoning, and Parmesan cheese. Dot with 2 tablespoons diet margarine and sprinkle with lemon juice. Bake uncovered for 35 minutes or until the fish is done in an oven set at 350 degrees. *Serves 4.*

CALORIES: 192.9
PROTEIN: 23.1 gm.
CARBOHYDRATE: 3.5 gm.
FAT: 8.9 gm.

CALCIUM: 168.7 mg.
SODIUM: 292 mg.
CHOLESTEROL: 90 mg.

Crab Imperial

8 ounces crabmeat
1 egg, beaten
3 tablespoons diet mayonnaise
2 teaspoons lemon juice
1/8 teaspoon seafood seasoning
3 egg whites, beaten
2 tablespoons diet mayonnaise
1/2 teaspoon lemon juice

In a mixing bowl combine the crabmeat, beaten egg, 3 tablespoons diet mayonnaise, 2 teaspoons lemon juice, and seafood seasoning. Blend well. Place in an oven set at 350 degrees and bake uncovered for 12 minutes. Meanwhile, beat the egg whites until they are stiff. Beat the 2 tablespoons diet mayonnaise with 1/2 teaspoon lemon juice and fold into the egg whites. Carefully spread the topping over the crabmeat. Return to the oven and bake 8 minutes until the topping is browned and puffed.
Serves 4.

CALORIES: 168.6
PROTEIN: 23.88 gm.
CARBOHYDRATE: 1.16 gm.
FAT: 3.56 gm.

CALCIUM: 58.12 mg.
SODIUM: 132 mg.
CHOLESTEROL: 153 mg.

Stuffed Green Peppers with Tuna

4 large green peppers
7 ounces water-packed tuna
1 tablespoon diet margarine
1/2 cup chopped onion
1/4 cup sliced celery
1/2 cup bean sprouts
5 ounces cream of celery soup
1/2 cup sliced cabbage
2 teaspoons soy sauce
1 egg, slightly beaten
2 tablespoons cracker crumbs
1 1/2 ounces Canadian style bacon, chopped
1/4 teaspoon pepper

Cut the tops off the green peppers and reserve. Clean the seeds out of the peppers. In a large saucepan, bring 8 cups of water to a boil and drop the peppers and their tops into the boiling water. Cook 5 minutes. Remove from the water and cool. Meanwhile, in a large mixing bowl combine the remaining ingredients. Blend well. Spoon into the green peppers. Place in a baking dish and bake 45 minutes in an oven set at 350 degrees.
Serves 4.

CALORIES: 201
PROTEIN: 18.6 gm.
CARBOHYDRATE: 14 gm.
FAT: 5.3 gm.

CALCIUM: 55.1 mg.
SODIUM: 790 mg.
CHOLESTEROL: 74.1 mg.

Shrimp Scampi

    3 tablespoons diet margarine
    1/4 cup sliced green onions
    1/2 cup mushrooms, sliced
    2 cloves garlic, minced
    1/2 teaspoon thyme
    2 tablespoons minced parsley
    1/2 teaspoon dry mustard
    1 1/2 pounds shrimp
    1/4 cup brandy

In a skillet, melt the diet margarine. Add the green onions, mushrooms, garlic, thyme, parsley, and dry mustard. Sauté 8 minutes over medium-high heat. Add the shrimp and cook 4 minutes until the shrimp turns pink. Pour in the brandy and set aflame. When the flames go out, serve.
Serves 4.

CALORIES: 223.9
PROTEIN: 42.1 gm.
CARBOHYDRATE: 4.6 gm.
FAT: 6.5 gm.

CALCIUM: 31.8 mg.
SODIUM: 4 mg.
CHOLESTEROL: 270 mg.

Seafood Cocktail

   2 ounces cooked crabmeat
   4 ounces cooked shrimp
   2 tablespoons lime juice
   ¼ cup seafood cocktail sauce
   Lettuce leaves

In a small mixing bowl combine the cooked crabmeat, cooked shrimp, lime juice, and 2 tablespoons of the seafood cocktail sauce. Blend the ingredients together. Add the remaining sauce if desired and chill 1 hour. Before serving line the serving bowl with lettuce leaves and divide the ingredients into 4 portions. Fill the serving bowl and top with a wedge of lime.
Serves 4.

CALORIES: 70.5   CALCIUM: 33 mg.
PROTEIN: 9.9 gm.   SODIUM: 201 mg.
CARBOHYDRATE: 5.8 gm.   CHOLESTEROL: 68 mg.
FAT: .8 gm.

Baked Red Snapper with Melon

   1 tomato, chopped
   1 onion, chopped
   2 cloves garlic
   2 tablespoons diet margarine
   1 tablespoon lemon juice
   5 drops hot pepper sauce
   1 tablespoon minced parsley
   4 4-ounce fillets of red snapper
   1 cantaloupe, cut into pieces

Put the tomato, onion, garlic, diet margarine, lemon juice, hot pepper sauce, and minced parsley in a small saucepan. Cook 5 minutes. Spread on each fillet. Place the fillets in a baking dish and bake 25 minutes or until the fish is done in an oven set at 350 degrees. Put the cantaloupe slices in a baking dish and place under the broiler until just brown on the edges. Serve alongside the fish.
Serves 4.

CALORIES: 221.3   CALCIUM: 74.2 mg.
PROTEIN: 23.5 gm.   SODIUM: 219 mg.
CARBOHYDRATE: 22.5 gm. CHOLESTEROL: 84 mg.
FAT: 18.7 gm.

Baked Fillet of Sole

1 1/2 pounds fillet of sole
2 tablespoons diet margarine
1/2 cup grated onion
2 cloves garlic, chopped
1/2 cup water
1 teaspoon dry mustard
2 teaspoons lemon juice
1 tablespoon Worcestershire sauce
1/4 teaspoon paprika
1 teaspoon soy sauce
1 tablespoon brown sugar
1/4 teaspoon white pepper
6 drops Tabasco sauce
3 tablespoons chopped parsley

Place the fillet of sole in a baking dish and set aside. In a saucepan, melt the margarine and stir in the grated onions and garlic. Sauté for 5 minutes. Add the remaining ingredients and bring to a boil over medium-high heat. Turn down the heat and simmer 30 minutes or until sauce is reduced by half. Pour over the fish. Place in an oven set at 350 degrees and bake uncovered for 35 minutes or until fish is flaky.

Serves 4.

CALORIES: 165
PROTEIN: 9.5 gm.
CARBOHYDRATE: 1.6 gm.
FAT: 3.7 gm.

CALCIUM: 10.5 mg.
SODIUM: 428 mg.
CHOLESTEROL: 126 mg.

18

Meats

Red meats like beef, pork, veal, lamb, and most game meats are high in marbleized fat and loaded with calories. Actually, it is the *invisible* fat—not the fat that you can trim off—that is the culprit. Whether preparing food for yourself, going to a restaurant, or going to a friend's home for dinner, you must try to stay away from red meat. If, however, red meat is the only choice, then request a portion of 3 to 4 ounces only. Every restaurant has a scale in the kitchen and the management should respect your wishes. Further, after a week on this diet, you should be able to figure out the correct amount just by looking.

If you have been a big meat eater, you will probably miss not having very much meat. I predict that after awhile you won't even want it anymore. You'll realize that it always leaves you feeling bloated and full. Besides, once you know how much it costs in calories, it really isn't worth it, is it?

When ordering, don't be fooled into thinking that if you order a casserole-style meat entrée such as stews or Stroganoffs you will avoid the nasty calories. Nine times out of ten those dishes are loaded with butter and cream, and your entire purpose will be defeated. Beware, beware! If you must have meat, shish kabob is a good choice. Be sure that whatever you order is only broiled or baked and has been prepared without added fats.

People who like eating meat often argue that it is the best source of protein. Of course, you should be an intelligent dieter and be certain that you get all the protein you would normally get when not dieting. But you can get just as much protein from fish as you can from calorie-laden red meat. I have included it in these menus only because I don't believe in giving up any one food group just to lose weight. So eat your meat dishes, but be careful to limit your intake.

BEEF

London Broil

1 onion, sliced
3 tablespoons beef bouillon
1 teaspoon Worcestershire sauce
2 cloves garlic, minced
$1/4$ teaspoon pepper
16 ounces London Broil

Place the onion, beef bouillon, Worcestershire sauce, garlic, and pepper in a small saucepan and heat through. Spread on top of the meat. Place the meat in a roasting pan and broil 5 minutes. Turn meat and broil an additional 5 minutes or until done. To serve, cut into thin slices cut on the angle.
Serves 4.

CALORIES: 232.8
PROTEIN: 35 gm.
CARBOHYDRATE: 2.4 gm.
FAT: 8.3 gm.

CALCIUM: 22.7 mg.
SODIUM: 120 mg.
CHOLESTEROL: 108 mg.

Gibson's Loaf

    1 tablespoon green pepper
    1 pound lean ground beef
    ¼ cup minced onion
    1 teaspoon poultry seasoning
    ¼ cup grated carrot
    ⅛ teaspoon pepper
    ¼ teaspoon paprika
    ¼ teaspoon chili powder
    1 egg, beaten
    ¼ cup milk
    ¼ cup dry bread crumbs

Mince the green pepper. Put the remaining ingredients into a mixing bowl and blend well. Place in a loaf pan and bake 1 hour at 350 degrees or until meat is done. Cool. Refrigerate. Slice into 8 portions.
Serves 8.

CALORIES: 122.5
PROTEIN: 13.1 gm.
CARBOHYDRATE: 1.6 gm.
FAT: 5.3 gm.

CALCIUM: 23.8 mg.
SODIUM: 72 mg.
CHOLESTEROL: 86 mg.

Salisbury Steak and Mushrooms

    4 3-ounce lean New York steaks
    Dash black pepper
    Dash garlic powder
    ½ cup beef broth
    2 tablespoons grated onion
    ⅛ cup red wine
    1 cup sliced mushrooms
    1 tablespoon diet margarine

Sprinkle the black pepper and garlic powder over the steaks. Broil the steaks to the desired doneness. Meanwhile, in a small saucepan, melt the diet margarine. Add the onions and sliced mushrooms and saute 4 minutes. Pour in the red wine and the beef broth. Bring the mixture to a boil. Reduce the heat and simmer 30 minutes. Serve over the steaks.

Serves 4.

CALORIES: 276
PROTEIN: 16 gm.
CARBOHYDRATE: 2.5 gm.
FAT: 22.5 gm.

CALCIUM: 9.8 mg.
SODIUM: 162 mg.
CHOLESTEROL: 56 mg.

VEAL

Roast Loin of Veal

    2 pounds loin of veal
    3 tablespoons lime juice
    3 tablespoons lemon juice
    1 teaspoon Worcestershire sauce
    1 teaspoon rosemary
    ½ teaspoon thyme
    ¼ teaspoon pepper

Make a basting sauce with the lime juice, lemon juice, Worcestershire sauce, rosemary, thyme, and pepper. Place the veal in a roasting pan on a rack. Place in an oven preheated to 325 degrees. Baste with the sauce. Roast 1 hour or until meat is done.

Serves 6.

CALORIES: 195
PROTEIN: 22.8 gm.
CARBOHYDRATE: 1.1 gm.
FAT: 103 gm.

CALCIUM: 13.5 mg.
SODIUM: 78 mg.
CHOLESTEROL: 144 mg.

Veal Marsala

1 pound veal cutlets, pounded
2 tablespoons flour
1/4 teaspoon white pepper
Vegetable cooking spray
2 tablespoons minced parsley
1 tablespoon diet margarine
1/2 cup dry Marsala wine
1 teaspoon lemon juice
Lemon wedges

Pound the cutlets very thin with a meat mallet. Dredge the meat in the flour, which has been seasoned with white pepper. Spray a skillet with vegetable cooking spray and in it melt the diet margarine. Sprinkle with the parsley. Place the cutlets in the skillet and cook over medium heat until browned on both sides. Add the Marsala and lemon juice and cook 1 minute. Serve with lemon wedges.

Serves 4.

CALORIES: 217
PROTEIN: 41.3 gm.
CARBOHYDRATE: 3.6 gm.
FAT: 9.7 gm.

CALCIUM: 26.4 mg.
SODIUM: 53 mg.
CHOLESTEROL: 108 mg.

LAMB

Lamb Shish Kabob

10 ounces lean lamb, cut into 8 pieces
2 tomatoes, cut in half
1 green pepper, cut in 4 pieces
1 large onion, quartered
4 large mushrooms
1/4 cup red wine
1/3 cup chopped green onions
4 cloves garlic, minced

Place 2 pieces of meat, 1 half tomato, 1 piece of green pepper, 1 piece of onion, and 1 mushroom on each skewer. In a mixing bowl make the marinade by combining the red wine, green onions, and minced garlic. Place kabobs in a shallow baking dish and pour the marinade over them. Marinate in the refrigerator 4 hours, turning every hour. Place kabobs under broiler and broil 4 inches from the heat, turning once. Broil until meat is done as desired. *Serves 4.*

CALORIES: 220
PROTEIN: 22 gm.
CARBOHYDRATE: 7 gm.
FAT: 10 gm.

CALCIUM: 26 mg.
SODIUM: 41 mg.
CHOLESTEROL: 68 mg.

Broiled Lamb Chops

1 tablespoon diet margarine, melted
2 cloves garlic, minced
2 tablespoons minced Chinese parsley
2 tablespoons rosé wine
4 5-ounce lamb chops
Ground pepper

In a small mixing bowl combine the margarine, garlic, parsley, and rosé wine. Brush the lamb chops with the spread and sprinkle liberally with ground pepper. Place chops in a pan on a rack and broil 12 minutes per side until chops are done. *Serves 4*

CALORIES: 140
PROTEIN: 20.9 gm.
CARBOHYDRATE: 1.4 gm.
FAT: 28 gm.

CALCIUM: 11.8 mg.
SODIUM: 90 mg.
CHOLESTEROL: 135 mg.

Leg of Lamb

½ leg of lamb (3 pounds)
3 cloves garlic
¼ cup parsley leaves
2 tablespoons water
1 tablespoon salad oil
2 teaspoons wine vinegar

Trim all visible fat from the leg of lamb. In a food processor fitted with a steel blade, combine the garlic, parsley leaves, water, oil, and vinegar. Whirl until well blended. Rub the parsley mixture into the lamb. Place the lamb in a roasting pan. Set the oven at 275 degrees and roast the lamb uncovered for 4 hours. Remove from oven and allow to sit for 15 minutes. Slice into thin slices.

Serves 4 5-ounce servings.

CALORIES: 145.2
PROTEIN: 16.8 gm.
CARBOHYDRATE: 2.4 gm.
FAT: 7.4 gm.

CALCIUM: 58 mg.
SODIUM: 91 mg.
CHOLESTEROL: 135 mg.

PORK

Pork Tenderloin

1 cup mushrooms, sliced
3 cloves garlic, minced
¼ cup green onions, chopped
1 tablespoon diet margarine
¼ teaspoon white pepper
¼ teaspoon thyme
¼ teaspoon oregano
½ cup chicken bouillon
12 ounces whole pork tenderloin

In a skillet, sauté the mushrooms, garlic, and green onions in the melted diet margarine. Stir in the seasonings. Cook over low heat for 5 minutes. Add the chicken bouillon. Place the meat in a baking

dish and pour the mushroom marinade over the meat. Roast at 450
degrees for 10 minutes or until done.
Serves 4.

CALORIES: 248 CALCIUM: 16.5 mg.
PROTEIN: 27 gm. SODIUM: 175 mg.
CARBOHYDRATE: 3.2 gm. CHOLESTEROL: 81 mg.
FAT: 14 gm.

Veal and Ham Terrine

This recipe is so simple. It's just like making meat loaf.

    8 ounces ground veal
    4 ounces ground ham
    ⅓ cup diet sour cream
    1 teaspoon thyme
    2 eggs, beaten
    2 ounces Cognac
    2 tablespoons minced onion
    1 clove garlic, minced
    1 ounce ground pork fat
    ¼ teaspoon pepper
    4 strips bacon
    2 ounces sliced ham
    12 pistachio nuts

Combine all the ingredients except the bacon strips, ham slices,
and nuts. Put into a food processor and blend until smooth. Put 2
of the bacon strips into a terrine mold and top with half the filling.
Lay the ham slices down the terrine lengthwise. Between the rows
of ham strips put the pistachio nuts. Top with the remaining
filling. Cover with the remaining 2 strips of bacon. Cover and put
into an oven set at 350 degrees. Bake 1½ hours or until the terrine
is done and remove from oven. Meanwhile, cover a brick with foil.
Remove cover from terrine and weight down terrine with the brick.
Chill. Refrigerate several days before serving.
Makes 12 slices.

CALORIES: 96.6 CALCIUM: 10.4 mg.
PROTEIN: 9.3 gm. SODIUM: 48 mg.
CARBOHYDRATE: 19 gm. CHOLESTEROL: 82 mg.
FAT: 7 gm.

19

Poultry

Poultry is not as fattening as meat. But the advice about eating meat also holds for eating poultry—stick to 3 or 4 ounces per serving. Also, when you are dining out, order it baked or broiled and be certain that it has been prepared without added fats. Always remove the skin before eating poultry because that is where most of the calories are found.

One important point: You can substitute rabbit in every chicken recipe and save yourself a few more calories. Rabbit is not eaten as much in America as it is in other countries. Though it is available every day in nearly every supermarket, it is often overlooked. It is usually packaged dressed and whole. Cut it into six pieces. From 1 pound of rabbit you will get about 8½ ounces of meat, which is a little better yield than from chicken. You can figure 61 calories per ounce for rabbit and 104 per ounce for chicken.

The midshipmen really gave me a hard time about rabbit being in their diet: "But we can't eat Thumper!" I could tell that their feelings ran deep, but believe me their fat cells ran deeper. The Thumper jokes finally disappeared. You, too, will find rabbit a satisfying addition to your diet.

Chicken Cashew

12 ounces chicken breast, meat only
1 tablespoon sherry
1 teaspoon soy sauce
1 clove garlic, minced
1 tablespoon cornstarch
¼ cup chicken bouillon
½ cup chopped onions
¼ cup chopped red bell pepper
¼ cup chopped green bell pepper
½ cup sliced celery
½ cup peas
½ ounce cashew nuts

Slice the chicken into strips. In a mixing bowl put the sherry, soy sauce, minced garlic, and cornstarch. Marinate the chicken pieces in this mixture and set aside. Arrange the other ingredients on a platter. Heat a wok and over high heat pour in the chicken bouillon. If the food items are to be properly cooked, it is important to heat the bare wok first and then add the broth (or when making regular Oriental dishes, the oil). This method prevents food from sticking to the bottom of the wok.

Drop the chicken into the wok and cook several minutes or until the chicken is done. Add the onion and green and red peppers. Then add the celery and peas and heat through. Toss with the cashew nuts. Add a little more soy sauce as needed.

Serves 4.

CALORIES: 134.2
PROTEIN: 20.1 gm.
CARBOHYDRATE: 8.2 gm.
FAT: 1.42 gm.

CALCIUM: 13.9 mg.
SODIUM: 375 mg.
CHOLESTEROL: 69 mg.

Baked Herbed Chicken

4 3½-ounce boned chicken breasts
4 teaspoons diet margarine
½ teaspoon paprika
⅛ teaspoon white pepper
1 teaspoon thyme
Pinch garlic powder
2 teaspoons lemon juice
½ cup chicken bouillon

Remove the skin from the chicken breasts. Place breasts in a glass baking dish. Spread each breast with 1 teaspoon of the diet margarine. Then sprinkle each with the paprika, white pepper, thyme, and garlic powder. Squeeze the lemon juice over the breasts. Pour the bouillon into the baking dish. Bake in the oven at 350 degrees for 25 minutes or until chicken is done.
Serves 4.

CALORIES: 173
PROTEIN: 26 gm.
CARBOHYDRATE: 5.3 gm.
FAT: 4.4 gm.

CALCIUM: 9.1 mg.
SODIUM: 120 mg.
CHOLESTEROL: 81 mg.

20

Desserts

"**B**ut will we get any desserts?" This was the first question every midshipman asked upon entering our Diet Room. You would have thought we were taking away their birthdays.

I knew that if the diet was going to be successful I would have to include enough sweets to satisfy these young adults. In this regard, the melon recipes were really helpful. They added "something sweet" to every meal without adding many calories. The versatile melon could be added to basic dessert recipes for variety. It's beautiful and delicious and offers the perfect ending to any meal, even if you're not on a diet. You'll find that melon is one part of the Annapolis Diet that will become a lifetime habit.

The midshipmen were on this diet at the Academy from Monday morning through Friday night. Saturday and Sunday they were left to home-cooked meals at officers' or sponsors' homes. They all commented on Monday mornings that they had had trouble keeping away from the sweets. Every Monday when I would weigh them I could tell which ones had gone on a sweet binge and which ones had not. The favorite excuse was "My sponsor tried out a new recipe for chocolate fudge and I just had to have some." My guess was that the sponsor made two batches: one for the midshipman and one for the rest of the family! The usual weekend weight gain was 2 pounds, and it would take until Wednesday for most mids to return to the weight they were before their binge. Sound familiar?

These recipes will help ease you through this seemingly impossible time. At the end of the diet you can splurge with a double fudge pie, if you still want it.

Soufflé Base

This basic recipe can be used to make numerous desserts. It is simple to make. It can be made ahead of time and frozen or simply made earlier in the day.

> 1 tablespoon diet margarine
> 1 tablespoon flour
> 1/4 cup 2 percent milk
> 1 cup cottage cheese
> 1 teaspoon lo-cal sweetener
> 1 egg yolk
> 2 teaspoons vanilla
> 6 egg whites

Make a white sauce: Melt the margarine in a saucepan and stir in the flour. Add the milk and heat over medium heat until thickened. Cool. In a food processor fitted with a steel blade, whirl the white sauce with the cottage cheese, lo-cal sweetener, egg yolk, and vanilla. Beat the egg whites until stiff. Use as a base for the soufflé recipes in this book.
Serves 8.

CALORIES: 85.3
PROTEIN: 9.5 gm.
CARBOHYDRATE: 3.03 gm.
FAT: 3.7 gm.

CALCIUM: 57.2 mg.
SODIUM: 102 mg.
CHOLESTEROL: 34.6 mg.

Apple Sweet

    Vegetable cooking spray
    2 apples, peeled and sliced
    1/4 cup lo-cal pancake mix
    1 packet lo-cal sweetener
    1/2 cup water
    1/2 teaspoon cinnamon
    1/8 teaspoon nutmeg
    1/2 cup apple juice

Spray a small oval baking dish with vegetable cooking spray. Place the sliced apples in the bottom of the dish. In a small mixing bowl, blend the pancake mix, sweetener, water, cinnamon, and nutmeg. When blended, add the apple juice. Pour over the sliced apples and bake in an oven set at 350 degrees. Bake for 20 minutes or until the batter is set.
Serves 4.

CALORIES: 72.9   CALCIUM: 7.9 mg.
PROTEIN: .75 gm.   SODIUM: 14.2 mg.
CARBOHYDRATE: 14.58 gm. CHOLESTEROL: 0 mg.
FAT: .43 gm.

Broiled Grapefruit

    1/4 teaspoon lo-cal sweetener
    1 teaspoon brown sugar
    2 grapefruit

Combine the lo-cal sweetener and brown sugar. Cut the grapefruit in half and remove the seeds. Cut along the membranes to loosen the sections. Sprinkle with the sugar mixture. Place under the broiler for 5 to 10 minutes or until the grapefruit bubbles and it is slightly browned.
Serves 4.

CALORIES: 175   CALCIUM: 60 mg.
PROTEIN: 2.0 gm.   SODIUM: 1 mg.
CARBOHYDRATE: 37.6 gm. CHOLESTEROL: 0 mg.
FAT: .4 gm.

Hot Fruit Compote

   1 apple
   1 orange
   8 plums
   1 cup reserved plum juice
   ½ cup apple juice
   Pinch nutmeg
   1 2-inch piece cinnamon stick
   Pinch cloves
   1 cup melon balls

Cut the apple into quarters. Peel and slice the orange. Drain the canned plums and reserve the liquid. Combine the plum juice, apple juice, and spices in a small saucepan and simmer 3 minutes. Stir in the apples, oranges, and plums and remove from the heat. Place in a baking dish and bake in an oven set at 300 degrees for 15 minutes. Stir in the melon balls. Serve in small glass dishes.
Serves 4.

CALORIES: 101.1
PROTEIN: 1 gm.
CARBOHYDRATE: 24.3 gm.
FAT: .4 gm.

CALCIUM: 30.5 mg.
SODIUM: 12.5 mg.
CHOLESTEROL: 0 mg.

Karen's Oranges

   4 large oranges, sliced
   2 tablespoons honey
   Fresh mint sprigs

Peel the orange so that none of the white membrane is left on the orange. Slice. Layer the slices in a bowl and pour the honey over them. Chill 2 hours. Turn the slices in the honey and juice that will have leached from the oranges. Chill another hour. Serve cold and garnish with sprigs of fresh mint.
Serves 4.

CALORIES: 128
PROTEIN: 2.35 gm.
CARBOHYDRATE: 8.20 gm.
FAT: .3 gm.

CALCIUM: 78 mg.
SODIUM: 1 mg.
CHOLESTEROL: 0 mg.

Lemon Custard

   1 egg, beaten
   1 teaspoon lo-cal sweetener

½ cup water
1 teaspoon unflavored gelatin
½ cup 2 percent milk
½ teaspoon vanilla extract
½ teaspoon lemon extract
2 teaspoons grated lemon peel

Beat the egg with the lo-cal sweetener. Bring the ½ cup water to a boil and dissolve the gelatin. In a saucepan, heat the milk and add the dissolved gelatin and bring to a boil. Stir in the egg and cook over medium heat, stirring until the custard thickens. Remove from the heat and stir in the vanilla extract and lemon extract. Stir in the lemon peel. Pour into custard cups and refrigerate.
Option: Substitute almond extract for the lemon extract and peel for Almond Custard.
Serves 4.

CALORIES: 38.25   CALCIUM: 46 mg.
PROTEIN: 4.71 gm.   SODIUM: 34 mg.
CARBOHYDRATE: 1.7 gm. CHOLESTEROL: 65.1 mg.
FAT: 1.4 gm.

Raspberry Parfait

1 ½ teaspoons unflavored gelatin
3 tablespoons orange juice
10 ounces raspberries
½ teaspoon lo-cal sweetener
1 cup plain yogurt

Soften the gelatin in the orange juice. Whirl the raspberries and the lo-cal sweetener in a food processor fitted with a steel blade. Stir the raspberry puree into the gelatin-orange juice mixture. Pour into a glass dish and refrigerate until set. Put the yogurt into the food processor and whirl until fluffy and light. Whip the set gelatin mixture with a whisk and fold in the yogurt. Spoon into champagne glasses.
Serves 6.

CALORIES: 51.6   CALCIUM: 5.67 mg.
PROTEIN: 2.65 gm.   SODIUM: 21.1 mg.
CARBOHYDRATE: 8.2 gm. CHOLESTEROL: 2.5 mg.
FAT: .74 gm.

Chocolate Mousse

This mousse is light and airy and only 53 calories.

    2 ounces sweet chocolate
    2 tablespoons diet margarine
    3 packets lo-cal sweetener
    1 tablespoon hot water
    1 teaspoon instant decaffeinated coffee
    1 tablespoon brandy
    1 whole egg
    ¼ cup dessert topping
    6 egg whites

In the top of a double boiler, melt the chocolate, diet margarine, and 2 packets of lo-cal sweetener. Stir in the hot water and instant coffee and brandy. Beat the whole egg slightly and then stir into the chocolate mixture. Cool the chocolate over ice. Meanwhile, beat the whipped topping according to package directions until it is stiff. Then beat the egg whites until stiff, and pour in the remaining packet of lo-cal sweetener. Carefully fold the dessert topping and the egg whites into the chocolate mixture. Pour into serving dishes and refrigerate overnight.
Serves 6.

CALORIES: 53.6   CALCIUM: 10.6 mg.
PROTEIN: 4.6 gm.   SODIUM: 61.1 mg.
CARBOHYDRATE: .55 gm.   CHOLESTEROL: 42.1 mg.
FAT: 3.51 gm.

Strawberry Mousse

    2 cups sliced strawberries
    5 egg whites
    ⅛ teaspoon cream of tartar
    2 packets lo-cal sweetener
    ½ teaspoon lemon juice
    ½ cup nondairy whipped topping

In a food processor fitted with a steel blade, whirl 1 cup of the strawberries until pureed. Reserve the remaining cup of strawber-

ries. Beat the egg whites and cream of tartar until the egg whites are stiff. Place the crushed strawberries in a mixing bowl and add the lo-cal sweetener and lemon juice. Carefully fold in the nondairy dessert topping and then fold in the remaining cup of sliced strawberries. Fold in the egg whites. Spoon into serving dishes. Refrigerate.
Serves 6.

CALORIES: 62.4
PROTEIN: 3.5 gm.
CARBOHYDRATE: 8.7 gm.
FAT: 1.4 gm.

CALCIUM: 3.5 mg.
SODIUM: 40.3 mg.
CHOLESTEROL: 0 mg.

Vanilla Sherbet

1 cup whole milk
1 envelope unflavored gelatin
1 cup buttermilk
2 teaspoons vanilla extract
1 teaspoon lo-cal sweetener
1 teaspoon grated lemon rind
1 egg white, beaten

Place the milk in a saucepan and bring to a boil. Remove from heat. Sprinkle the gelatin over the milk and stir until the gelatin is dissolved. Add the buttermilk, vanilla extract, lo-cal sweetener, and lemon rind. Fold in the egg white. Pour into a jelly roll pan and place in the freezer until firm. Remove from freezer, whip the mixture, and return to the freezer. Repeat twice. Remove from freezer and serve with an ice cream scoop.
Serves 6.

CALORIES: 44.1
PROTEIN: 2.3 gm.
CARBOHYDRATE: 4.7 gm.
FAT: 1.4 gm.

CALCIUM: 94.7 mg.
SODIUM: 73.4 mg.
CHOLESTEROL: 9 mg.

Baked Pears in Melon

⅛ teaspoon cinnamon
Dash mace
1 tablespoon flour
1 tablespoon diet margarine
1 tablespoon lemon juice
2 packets lo-cal sweetener
8 slices cantaloupe
3 cups sliced pears

Mix the spices and the flour. Melt the diet margarine, lemon juice, and sweetener, and stir into the flour mixture. Put the cantaloupe slices in the bottom of a glass baking dish and top with the sliced pears. Pour the flour mixture over all and bake for 15 minutes in an oven set at 350 degrees.
Serves 6.

CALORIES: 67.5
PROTEIN: .7 gm.
CARBOHYDRATE: 14.8 gm.
FAT: 1.3 gm.

CALCIUM: 12.7 mg.
SODIUM: 10.6 mg.
CHOLESTEROL: 0 mg.

Blueberry Melon Fluff

5 ounces blueberries
1 teaspoon unflavored gelatin
1 tablespoon cold water
2 egg whites
½ teaspoon lo-cal sweetener
1 teaspoon vanilla
½ teaspoon lemon juice
1 teaspoon grated lemon rind
¼ cup diet whipped topping
1 cup melon balls

Place the blueberries in a food processor fitted with a steel blade and whirl until the fruit is pureed. Soften the gelatin in the cold water and then dissolve over a pan of hot water. Beat the egg whites until frothy. Place in the bowl of an electric mixer. Beat until very stiff. In a mixing bowl, combine the pureed blueberries, lo-cal sweetener, vanilla, lemon juice, and lemon rind. Fold the blueberry mixture into the stiff egg whites. Fold in the whipped diet dessert topping. Pour into champagne glasses and chill. Serve garnished with melon balls.

Serves 4.

CALORIES: 30.2 CALCIUM: 2 mg.
PROTEIN: 13.45 gm. SODIUM: 29 mg.
CARBOHYDRATE: 2.7 gm. CHOLESTEROL: 0 mg.
FAT: 1 gm.

Coconut Melon Custard

1 package instant diet vanilla pudding mix
1 teaspoon coconut extract
1 cup cantaloupe balls
$1/2$ ounce flaked coconut, toasted

Prepare the pudding mix according to package directions. Stir in the coconut extract and cantaloupe balls and pour into serving dishes. Top with the flaked coconut.

Serves 8.

CALORIES: 79.5 CALCIUM: 4.1 mg.
PROTEIN: 4.2 gm. SODIUM: 86.8 mg.
CARBOHYDRATE: 13.6 gm. CHOLESTEROL: 2 mg.
FAT: 3.6 gm.

Honeydew Whip

1 tablespoon unflavored gelatin
3 tablespoons diet ginger ale
1 cup mashed honeydew melon
2 packets lo-cal sweetener
3 egg whites
$1/2$ cup lo-cal dessert topping

Dissolve the gelatin in the diet ginger ale. Put the gelatin–ginger ale mixture, mashed melon, and sweetener in a small saucepan. Cook over medium heat until the mixture thickens. Remove from heat and cool. Whip the egg whites until they form stiff peaks. Carefully fold the egg whites into the melon mixture. Fold in the dessert topping. Chill.

Serves 4.

CALORIES: 64 CALCIUM: 18.2 mg.
PROTEIN: 5.4 gm. SODIUM: 42 mg.
CARBOHYDRATE: 5.5 gm. CHOLESTEROL: 0 mg.
FAT: 1.9 gm.

Melon Coconut Kabob

1 cup cantaloupe, cut into chunks
1 cup watermelon, cut into chunks
½ cup honeydew, cut into chunks
2 tablespoons orange juice
½ cup shredded coconut

Put alternating colors of melon pieces onto a wooden skewer. Sprinkle with orange juice and roll in coconut. Chill. *Serves 8.*

CALORIES: 44.6
PROTEIN: .6 gm.
CARBOHYDRATE: 4.8 gm.
FAT: 28.6 gm.

CALCIUM: 7.4 mg.
SODIUM: 6.1 mg.
CHOLESTEROL: 0 mg.

Orange Melon Parfait

1 ½ teaspoons unflavored gelatin
3 tablespoons orange juice
2 oranges, chopped
½ teaspoon lo-cal sweetener
1 cup plain yogurt
1 cup honeydew melon balls

Soften the gelatin in the orange juice. Whirl half the oranges and the lo-cal sweetener in a food processor fitted with a steel blade. Stir the orange puree into the gelatin-orange juice mixture. Pour into a glass dish and refrigerate until set. Put the yogurt into the food processor and whirl until fluffy and light. Whip the set gelatin mixture with a whisk and fold in the yogurt and remaining oranges. Fold in the honeydew melon balls. Spoon into champagne glasses. *Serves 6.*

CALORIES: 63.5
PROTEIN: 1.4 gm.
CARBOHYDRATE: 15.3 gm.
FAT: .3 gm.

CALCIUM: 24.5 mg.
SODIUM: 24.5 mg.
CHOLESTEROL: 2.5 mg.

Melon Freeze

1 cantaloupe
2 cups watermelon, cut into cubes
2 packets lo-cal sweetener
1/3 cup diet 7-Up

Cut the cantaloupe into quarters. Meanwhile, put the watermelon into the blender and whirl until mashed. Add the sweetener and the diet 7-Up. Pour the mixture into ice cube trays and freeze. (It is best to use the tiny ice cube trays.) To serve, put melon cubes on each piece of cantaloupe.
Serves 4.

CALORIES: 63.5
PROTEIN: 1.4 gm.
CARBOHYDRATE: 15.3 gm.
FAT: .3 gm.

CALCIUM: 24.5 mg.
SODIUM: 14.5 mg.
CHOLESTEROL: 0 mg.

Raspberry Melon Parfait

1 1/2 teaspoons unflavored gelatin
3 tablespoons orange juice
10 ounces raspberries
1/2 teaspoon lo-cal sweetener
1 cup plain yogurt
1 cup honeydew melon balls

Soften the gelatin in the orange juice. Whirl the raspberries and the lo-cal sweetener in a food processor fitted with a steel blade. Stir the raspberry puree into the gelatin-orange juice mixture. Pour into a glass dish and refrigerate until set. Put the yogurt into the food processor and whirl until fluffy and light. Whip the set gelatin mixture with a whisk and fold in the yogurt. Stir in the honeydew melon balls. Spoon into champagne glasses.
Serves 6.

CALORIES: 51.6
PROTEIN: 2.6 gm.
CARBOHYDRATE: 8.2 gm.
FAT: .7 gm.

CALCIUM: 5.7 mg.
SODIUM: 24.3 mg.
CHOLESTEROL: 0 mg.

Melon Grape Freeze

    ½ cantaloupe
    2 cups white grape juice
    10 ice cubes

Peel and seed the cantaloupe and cut into small cubes. Put the cantaloupe, grape juice, and ice cubes in a blender and frappé until the ingredients are well blended. Put in the freezer for 1 hour. Stir just before serving.
Serves 6.

CALORIES: 69.3   CALCIUM: 15.7 mg.
PROTEIN: .5 gm.   SODIUM: 6 mg.
CARBOHYDRATE: 17.4 gm.   CHOLESTEROL: 0 mg.
FAT: Trace

Watermelon Mousse

    2½ cups sliced strawberries
    5 egg whites
    ⅛ teaspoon cream of tartar
    2 packets lo-cal sweetener
    ½ teaspoon lemon juice
    ½ cup nondairy whipped topping
    2 cups watermelon balls

In a food processor fitted with a steel blade, whirl 1½ cups of the strawberries until they are crushed. Reserve the remaining cup of strawberries. Beat the egg whites and cream of tartar until the egg whites are stiff. Place the crushed strawberries in a mixing bowl and add the lo-cal sweetener and lemon juice. Carefully fold in the nondairy dessert topping, the remaining cup of sliced strawberries, and the melon balls. Fold in the egg whites. Spoon into serving dishes. Chill.
Serves 6.

CALORIES: 62.4   CALCIUM: 3.5 mg.
PROTEIN: 3.5 gm.   SODIUM: 41 mg.
CARBOHYDRATE: 8.7 gm.   CHOLESTEROL: 0 mg.
FAT: 1.4 gm.

21

Gourmet Recipes

Soups

Chicken Gumbo Soup

1 cup cooked chicken meat
2 tablespoons flour
2 tablespoons diet margarine
2 slices lo-cal bacon, chopped
1½ cups fresh okra
1 tomato, chopped
1 onion, chopped
2 cups chicken bouillon
3 cups water
1 bay leaf
1 clove garlic, minced
2 tablespoons parsley, minced
1 teaspoon filé powder
Dash pepper

Cut the chicken meat into pieces and sprinkle with flour. In a stockpot, melt the diet margarine and fry the chicken pieces until they are golden brown. Remove chicken. Add the chopped bacon, okra, tomato, and onion and fry. Add the remaining ingredients except the pepper. Cook for 2 hours. Season with pepper to taste. *Serves 6.*

CALORIES: 94.8
PROTEIN: 9.9 gm.
CARBOHYDRATE: 7.1 gm.
FAT: 3.4 gm.

CALCIUM: 47.5 mg.
SODIUM: 195 mg.
CHOLESTEROL: 32 mg.

French Onion Soup

    2 tablespoons diet margarine
    6 cups onions, sliced
    3 cloves garlic, minced
    3 tablespoons minced parsley
    4 cups beef bouillon
    2 cups chicken bouillon
    1 teaspoon Worcestershire sauce
    1/2 teaspoon coarse black pepper
    6 onion melba rounds
    1 ounce Swiss cheese, grated

In a saucepan, melt the diet margarine. Put in the onions, garlic, and parsley and sauté for 45 minutes. Cook until the onions are dark brown. Add the bouillon, Worcestershire sauce, and pepper. Heat through. Turn the heat down and simmer for 15 minutes. Pour into serving bowls and drop 1 onion round into each bowl. Sprinkle Swiss cheese over all and put under the broiler to melt the cheese.

Serves 12.

CALORIES: 45   CALCIUM: 36.5 mg.
PROTEIN: 2 gm.   SODIUM: 516 mg.
CARBOHYDRATE: 6.4 gm.   CHOLESTEROL: 3.7 mg.
FAT: 1.1 gm.

Lobster Bisque

    2 cups 2 percent milk
    1 cup clam juice
    1 cup chicken bouillon
    1/2 teaspoon paprika
    1/4 teaspoon onion powder
    White pepper
    1 egg, beaten
    1 1/2 cups cooked lobster meat

In a saucepan combine the milk, clam juice, chicken bouillon, and the seasonings. Bring to a boil. Stir in the beaten egg and cook

until slightly thickened. Add the lobster meat and heat through over low heat.
Serves 8.

CALORIES: 72
PROTEIN: 8.5 gm.
CARBOHYDRATE: 3.8 gm.
FAT: 2.5 gm.

CALCIUM: 109 mg.
SODIUM: 222 mg.
CHOLESTEROL: 103 mg.

Gazpacho

 2 cups tomato juice
 1 tomato, diced
 1/3 cup sliced cucumber
 3 tablespoons chopped green pepper
 1/4 cup chopped onion
 1/4 cup rosé wine
 2 tablespoons red wine vinegar
 1 clove garlic, minced
 1 cup beef bouillon
 Ground red pepper
 2 green chilies, chopped
 1/2 teaspoon Worcestershire sauce
 Juice of 1/2 lemon
 Black pepper

Combine all the ingredients in a glass bowl. Refrigerate. Serve chilled.
Serves 4.

CALORIES: 47.5
PROTEIN: 1.9 gm.
CARBOHYDRATE: 11.02 gm.
FAT: .05 gm.

CALCIUM: 7.05 mg.
SODIUM: 255 mg.
CHOLESTEROL: 0 mg.

Tortilla Soup

¼ cup chopped onion
¼ cup tomato soup
2 tablespoons diet catsup
1 tomato, chopped
6 cups chicken broth
2 green chilies, chopped
1 tablespoon Chinese parsley, chopped
1 cup tortilla chips
6 tablespoons Parmesan cheese

In a saucepan, combine all the ingredients except the tortilla chips and Parmesan cheese. Bring to a boil and then turn down the heat. Simmer for 30 minutes. To serve, pour into bowls and sprinkle with broken tortilla chips and a tablespoon of Parmesan cheese. Season with pepper to taste.
Serves 6.

CALORIES: 55
PROTEIN: 1.8 gm.
CARBOHYDRATE: 6.76 gm.
FAT: 2.48 gm.

CALCIUM: 7.73 mg.
SODIUM: 870 mg.
CHOLESTEROL: 7.5 mg.

Salads

Artichoke Salad

1 cup artichoke hearts
1 cup artichoke bottoms
1 tomato, sliced
1 avocado, chopped
1 onion, chopped
3 tablespoons diet French dressing

Place all the ingredients into a salad bowl and toss. Marinate in refrigerator 3 hours before serving.
Serves 4.

CALORIES: 130.75   CALCIUM: 32.5 mg.
PROTEIN: 2.8 gm.   SODIUM: 116 mg.
CARBOHYDRATE: 10.1 gm.   CHOLESTEROL: 0 mg.
FAT: 9.3 gm.

Bouillabaisse Salad

        8 ounces cooked shrimp
        8 ounces cooked lobster
        1 head iceberg lettuce
        1/2 head Romaine lettuce
        4 tomatoes
        8 ounces cooked fillet of sole
        8 ounces crabmeat
        3 ounces diet French dressing
        1/4 cup chopped parsley
        1 red onion, sliced
        Lemon twists

Cut the shrimp in half and cut the lobster into bite-size pieces.
Break the lettuce into whole leaves to form lettuce bowls. Cut the
tomatoes into wedges and set aside. In a large mixing bowl combine
the shrimp, lobster, fillet of sole, and crabmeat. Pour the diet
French dressing over the seafood. Toss with the parsley. Sprinkle
the onion slices over all and mix well. Refrigerate 3 hours or
overnight. To serve, divide the mixture into 4 equal portions and
put into the lettuce bowls. Garnish with the tomato wedges and
lemon twists.
Serves 4.

CALORIES: 305   CALCIUM: 246.3 mg.
PROTEIN: 68.8 gm.   SODIUM: 221 mg.
CARBOHYDRATE: 15.4 gm.   CHOLESTEROL: 265 mg.
FAT: 3.5 gm.

Caesar Salad

- 2 cloves garlic, split
- 2 anchovy fillets
- ¼ cup lemon juice
- 2 tablespoons red wine vinegar
- ½ teaspoon black pepper
- 1 teaspoon Worcestershire sauce
- 1 coddled egg
- 1 head Romaine lettuce
- 1 ounce blue cheese, crumbled

Rub a wooden salad bowl with the split garlic. In the bowl, mash the anchovies and whisk in the lemon juice, wine vinegar, pepper, and Worcestershire sauce and beat in the coddled egg. Add the lettuce and toss. Sprinkle the crumbled blue cheese over the salad greens.

Serves 4.

Hint: Soak the anchovies in milk for 30 minutes before adding them to the recipe. Rinse off the milk with cold water and pat dry. Then add to the recipe. This will remove the oil and some of the salt that has been used as a preservative.

CALORIES: 71.8　　　　CALCIUM: 77 mg.
PROTEIN: 22 gm.　　　SODIUM: 35 mg.
CARBOHYDRATE: 4.8 gm.　CHOLESTEROL: 63 mg.
FAT: 5.9 gm.

Crab Pasta Salad

2 tablespoons diet mayonnaise
1 tablespoon lemon juice
3 tablespoons minced parsley
1/4 teaspoon pepper
2 tablespoons chopped pimiento
1/4 cup chopped green onion
1 teaspoon prepared mustard
1/4 teaspoon seafood seasoning
1 egg, beaten
1/4 cup yogurt
2 cups cooked macaroni shells
8 ounces cooked crabmeat

Put the diet mayonnaise, lemon juice, minced parsley, pepper, pimiento, green onion, mustard, seafood seasoning, egg, and yogurt into a mixing bowl and whisk together. Stir in the cooked shells and crabmeat. Toss and chill.
Serves 4.

CALORIES: 150.6
PROTEIN: 13.3 gm.
CARBOHYDRATE: 6.1 gm.
FAT: 15.6 gm.

CALCIUM: 91.5 mg.
SODIUM: 51 mg.
CHOLESTEROL: 113 mg.

Salade Niçoise

Dressing:

¾ cup beef bouillon
¼ cup wine vinegar
1 tablespoon lemon juice
¼ teaspoon garlic powder
¼ teaspoon ground pepper
3 tablespoons chopped chives
3 tablespoons minced parsley
¼ teaspoon onion powder

4 medium potatoes
1 10-ounce package frozen French green beans
1 head iceberg lettuce
1 large can tuna, packed in water
2 large tomatoes
2 hard-cooked eggs
4 boiling onions
8 ripe pitted olives
6 anchovy fillets

Prepare the dressing recipe first. Put all the ingredients in a glass jar and shake until blended. To prepare the salad, boil the potatoes in their jackets. When they are done remove from heat and pour off the water. Cool. Peel the potatoes and then dice them into ½-inch cubes. Put the potato cubes into a small saucepan and pour ½ of the dressing over them. Cook over medium heat for 5 minutes. Put the thawed green beans into a bowl and pour the remaining dressing over them. Cut the lettuce into bite-size pieces and arrange on a large serving platter. Drain the tuna and invert the can in the center of the serving platter on top of the bed of lettuce. Remove the potatoes from the marinade and arrange them around the tuna. Put the green beans around the potatoes. Cut the tomatoes into wedges and the eggs into slices and put around the green beans. Peel and slice the boiling onions into rings. Sprinkle them over the entire salad. Garnish the platter with pitted olives and with anchovy fillets that have been soaked in a little milk, then patted dry. Pour the remaining dressing from the potatoes and the green beans over all. Serve chilled.
Serves 12.

CALORIES: 95.7
PROTEIN: 8.3 gm.
CARBOHYDRATE: 11.5 gm.
FAT: 2 gm.

CALCIUM: 47 mg.
SODIUM: 76 mg.
CHOLESTEROL: 42 mg.

Chesapeake Bay Salad

1 cup shredded lettuce
2 ounces crabmeat
2 tablespoons diet mayonnaise
3 tablespoons sliced green onions
Dash seafood seasoning
1/4 avocado
3 large cooked shrimp
2 fresh oysters
1/2 tomato, cut into wedges
1/4 cantaloupe

Put the shredded lettuce on a serving plate. Put the crabmeat in a small mixing bowl. Moisten with the diet mayonnaise. Stir in the green onion slices and season with seafood seasoning. Blend well. Remove the skin from the avocado slice and lay on its side. Fill the avocado crescent with the crabmeat. Arrange the shrimp and the opened fresh oysters in the shell on the serving plate. Garnish with tomato wedges and cantaloupe slice.
Serves 1.

CALORIES: 92
PROTEIN: 1.2 gm.
CARBOHYDRATE: 3.2 gm.
FAT: 15.1 gm.

CALCIUM: 128.9 mg.
SODIUM: 642 mg.
CHOLESTEROL: 321 mg.

Rose Petal Melon Salad

1 head Boston lettuce
9 roses of various colors
½ cup sliced celery
2 cups cantaloupe balls
2 teaspoons honey
3 tablespoons orange juice

Clean the lettuce and break into pieces. Clean the roses and separate into petals. Discard the centers. Trim the petals of the bitter white portion at the base. Toss the petals and lettuce with the celery. Arrange on a serving platter. Garnish with additional petals and the melon balls. Combine the honey and orange juice and pour over the salad.
Serves 6.

CALORIES: 32.1   CALCIUM: 22.4 mg.
PROTEIN: .8 gm.   SODIUM: 22 mg.
CARBOHYDRATE: 7.8 gm.   CHOLESTEROL: 0 mg.
FAT: .1 gm.

Boston Melon Salad

1 cup cooked white chicken meat
1 orange
1 cup honeydew melon balls
½ cup sliced strawberries
¼ cup sliced green onion
1 ounce blue cheese, crumbled
2 tablespoons lime juice
3 tablespoons beef bouillon
Dash white pepper
4 cups Romaine lettuce, shredded

Remove the skin from the chicken meat and cut into cubes. Toss the chicken and fruit together in a salad bowl. Add the green onion slices and blue cheese. In a small mixing bowl whisk the lime juice and beef bouillon together and season with pepper. Add the lettuce to the chicken and fruits and drizzle the dressing over all. Toss lightly.
Serves 6.

CALORIES: 101.6
PROTEIN: 10.7 gm.
CARBOHYDRATE: 9.6 gm.
FAT: 2.1 gm.

CALCIUM: 60.2 mg.
SODIUM: 27 mg.
CHOLESTEROL: 229 mg.

Shrimp and Scallop Salad

24 large shrimp
1 pound scallops
1/2 pound Chinese snow peas
1 small cucumber, sliced
1/2 cup sliced celery
1/3 cup chicken bouillon
Water
1/3 cup white vinegar
2 tablespoons light soy sauce
2 teaspoons dry mustard
1/2 teaspoon sesame oil
2 tablespoons sherry
1 packet lo-cal sweetener

Cook the shrimp in water until it just turns pink. Cook the scallops in 1/2 cup water until translucent. Drain the seafood and cool. String the snow peas and submerge in boiling water for 30 seconds. Remove. Slice the cucumber. In a small mixing bowl, toss the snow peas and cucumber slices. Toss the celery slices with the seafood. Meanwhile, in a mixing bowl whisk the bouillon, water, vinegar, soy sauce, mustard, sesame oil, sherry, and lo-cal sweetener. Arrange the seafood in the center of a serving platter that has been lined with lettuce leaves. Put the snow peas and cucumbers around the seafood. Drizzle with dressing.
Serves 6.

CALORIES: 145
PROTEIN: 24.6 gm.
CARBOHYDRATE: 4.7 gm.
FAT: 2.3 gm.

CALCIUM: 139.6 mg.
SODIUM: 728 mg.
CHOLESTEROL: 466 mg.

Breads

Cheese Popovers

1 cup flour
1/4 teaspoon seafood seasoning
1 tablespoon Parmesan cheese
2 eggs, beaten
1/2 cup 2 percent milk
1/2 cup water
Vegetable cooking spray

In a large mixing bowl put the flour, seafood seasoning, and Parmesan cheese. Blend. Beat together the eggs, milk, and water and stir into the flour mixture, being careful not to overmix. Spray muffin cups with vegetable cooking spray and fill the cups two-thirds full. Place in the lower half of an oven set at 350 degrees. Bake 15 minutes or until browned and puffed.

Serves 8.

CALORIES: 93.3	CALCIUM: 65.75 mg.
PROTEIN: 38.3 gm.	SODIUM: 24 mg.
CARBOHYDRATE: 13.8 gm.	CHOLESTEROL: 66 mg.
FAT: 2.1 gm.	

Crêpes

2 eggs, beaten
1/2 cup 2 percent milk
1/2 cup water
1/2 cup flour

Whisk the ingredients in a mixing bowl. Let stand 15 minutes. Heat a 7-inch crêpe pan that is well seasoned and has been sprayed with vegetable cooking spray. Pour a quarter cup of batter at a time into the pan. Brown each crêpe on one side, then slip over to the other side and brown. Makes 16 7-inch crêpes.

Serves 16.

CALORIES: 22	CALCIUM: 12.94 mg.
PROTEIN: 1.32 gm.	SODIUM: 13.4 mg.
CARBOHYDRATE: 2.61 gm.	CHOLESTEROL: 32 mg.
FAT: .73 gm.	

Fruits

Apricot Melon Cup

2 small cantaloupes
1 cup honeydew melon balls
1 cup apricot halves
1/8 teaspoon ground cardamon

Cut the cantaloupes into halves and clean. Put the melon balls and apricots in a mixing bowl and stir in the cardamon. Fill the melon halves with the fresh fruit.
Serves 4.

CALORIES: 119.2
PROTEIN: 2.7 gm.
CARBOHYDRATE: 32.2 gm.
FAT: .5 gm.

CALCIUM: 17.3 mg.
SODIUM: 24 mg.
CHOLESTEROL: 0 mg.

Pineapple Melon Boat

1 pineapple
1 banana, sliced
1 tablespoon lemon juice
1 cup fresh strawberries
1/2 cup strawberry yogurt
2 tablespoons orange juice

Cut the pineapple in quarters and remove the core. Loosen the fruit and cut into sections, leaving them in place. Put the quarters on serving plates. Peel the banana and cut into slices. Dip the slices into the lemon juice to prevent the fruit from turning brown. Stem and clean the strawberries and slice them. Mix the strawberries and banana together and put on top of the pineapple. In a food processor fitted with a steel blade, whirl the strawberry yogurt and orange juice until well blended. Pour the dressing on top of the fruit boat. Put on serving plates.
Serves 6.

CALORIES: 68.7
PROTEIN: 1.2 gm.
CARBOHYDRATE: 15.3 gm.
FAT: .9 gm.

CALCIUM: 39.3 mg.
SODIUM: 22 mg.
CHOLESTEROL: 0 mg.

Eggs

Eggs Benedict
    1 English muffin
    2 eggs
    1 slice Canadian bacon
    4 tablespoons diet Hollandaise sauce, recipe below
    Dash white pepper
    Parsley to garnish

Toast the English muffin. Poach the eggs. Cut the Canadian bacon in half. Place half on each half of the English muffin. Top each half with a poached egg. Pour the Hollandaise sauce over all. Sprinkle with pepper and garnish with fresh parsley.
Serves 2.

CALORIES: 217
PROTEIN: 17.3 gm.
CARBOHYDRATE: 31.8 gm.
FAT: 9.1 gm.

CALCIUM: 40 mg.
SODIUM: 442.1 mg.
CHOLESTEROL: 338 mg.

Diet Hollandaise Sauce
    1 tablespoon diet margarine
    1 tablespoon flour
    1/2 cup 2 percent milk
    1/4 cup water
    2 egg yolks
    1 tablespoon lemon juice
    1/8 teaspoon white pepper

In a saucepan, melt the diet margarine and stir in the flour. Cook over medium heat for 3 minutes, stirring all the while. Pour in the milk and water. Stir with a whisk until the mixture is smooth. Beat the egg yolks and stir in the lemon juice and pepper. Pour into the sauce and whisk until smooth and thickened. One serving is 2 tablespoons.
Makes 1 cup.

CALORIES: 36
PROTEIN: .4 gm.
CARBOHYDRATE: .7 gm.
FAT: 1.5 gm.

CALCIUM: 3.4 mg.
SODIUM: 61 mg.
CHOLESTEROL: 253 mg.

Huevos Rancheros

1 tablespoon minced onion
1 clove garlic
1 tablespoon Chinese parsley
3 tablespoons finely chopped tomato
2 green chilies
1 tablespoon diet catsup
½ teaspoon oregano
Dash black pepper
4 ounces vegetable juice
1 corn tortilla
2 eggs

In a saucepan, combine the onion, garlic, parsley, tomato, chilies, catsup, oregano, pepper, and vegetable juice. Bring to a boil and simmer 15 minutes. In an oval baking dish, place the corn tortilla. Pour the sauce over the tortilla and break the 2 eggs into the sauce. Bake in an oven set at 325 degrees until the eggs are set.
Serves 1.

CALORIES: 248
PROTEIN: 13.3 gm.
CARBOHYDRATE: 3.0 gm.
FAT: 11 gm.

CALCIUM: 63 mg.
SODIUM: 380 mg.
CHOLESTEROL: 506 mg.

Ranchero Omelet

1 teaspoon diet margarine
3 tablespoons chopped green pepper
3 tablespoons chopped onion
3 tablespoons chopped tomato
2 large whole eggs
1 tablespoon diet catsup
1/2 teaspoon water
1/2 teaspoon oregano
Dash black pepper

In an 8-inch omelet pan, melt the diet margarine and add the green peppers, onion, and tomato. Sauté 4 minutes. Meanwhile, in a small mixing bowl beat the eggs with the remaining ingredients. When the vegetables are soft, pour the egg mixture over them. Make the omelet using the same technique as for the cheese omelet (see page 124). When eggs are set, turn out onto a serving platter.
Makes 1 omelet.

CALORIES: 196
PROTEIN: 13.6 gm.
CARBOHYDRATE: 7.6 gm.
FAT: 13 gm.

CALCIUM: 72 mg.
SODIUM: 140 mg.
CHOLESTEROL: 506 mg.

Western Omelet

½ tablespoon diet margarine
2 tablespoons minced onion
2 teaspoons minced green pepper
3 tablespoons chopped tomato
1½ ounces Canadian bacon
¼ teaspoon Worcestershire sauce
Dash pepper
2 eggs
1 teaspoon water

Melt the margarine in an omelet pan and sauté the onion, green pepper, tomato, and chopped Canadian bacon. Stir in the Worcestershire sauce and pepper. Remove from the pan and wipe pan clean. Keep the sauce mixture warm. Meanwhile, make an omelet with the eggs and water. Turn out onto a serving platter and top with the warm sauce.

Serves 2.

CALORIES: 161
PROTEIN: 12.6 gm.
CARBOHYDRATE: 9 gm.
FAT: 5.6 gm.

CALCIUM: 46 mg.
SODIUM: 883 mg.
CHOLESTEROL: 294 mg.

Casseroles

Moussaka Turkish Style
Vegetable cooking spray
2 eggplants
Salt
2 tablespoons water
1 pound ground lamb
¼ cup chopped onion
2 cloves garlic, minced
2 tablespoons Chinese parsley, chopped
½ teaspoon pepper
2 tomatoes, chopped
¼ cup chicken bouillon
Dash ground cloves
½ teaspoon oregano
¼ cup bread crumbs
¼ cup Parmesan cheese

Sauce:
1 onion, minced
2 cloves garlic, minced
¼ cup chopped green pepper
1 bay leaf
¼ teaspoon allspice
⅛ teaspoon pepper
2 tablespoons Chinese parsley
½ cup chicken bouillon

Spray a skillet with the vegetable cooking spray. Cut the eggplant in half lengthwise. Sprinkle with a little salt and allow to rest for 30 minutes. Pat dry with a paper towel. Run under cold water and pat dry again.

Sprinkle 2 tablespoons water over the eggplant in a pan and cover. Place over medium heat and cook until the vegetable is tender. Cool. Scoop out the flesh, being careful not to tear the skin. Set the skins aside and reserve the pulp.

Place the lamb, onions, garlic, and parsley in the skillet and sauté until the lamb is cooked. Add the remaining ingredients except for the Parmesan cheese and simmer 5 minutes. Meanwhile, chop the reserved eggplant pulp. Mix into the lamb mixture. Fill the eggplant with the lamb filling. Place the filled eggplant in a shallow baking dish and sprinkle with the Parmesan cheese. Bake for 45 minutes in a water bath in an oven set at 375 degrees. Meanwhile, prepare the sauce. In a skillet, simmer the other ingredients in the chicken bouillon over medium heat, stirring all the while. Reduce the heat to low and cook until thickened. Remove the eggplant from the oven and top with the sauce. Serve hot.
Serves 8.

CALORIES: 252.2
PROTEIN: 20 gm.
CARBOHYDRATE: 13.5 gm.
FAT: 13.1 gm.

CALCIUM: 135.1 mg.
SODIUM: 204 mg.
CHOLESTEROL: 86 mg.

Paella

    3 tablespoons diet margarine
    12 ounces chicken
    Flour
    1 onion, chopped
    1 tomato, chopped
    6 ounces lobster meat
    4 ounces shrimp
    3 ounces Canadian bacon, minced
    1 cup uncooked rice
    1½ cups peas
    2 cups chicken bouillon
    1 teaspoon paprika
    4 cloves garlic, minced
    3 tablespoons chili powder
    1 teaspoon saffron

Melt the diet margarine in a skillet. Dust the chicken with a little flour and sauté in the margarine. Remove from the pan and reserve. Add the chopped onion and tomato and sauté for 4 minutes. Stir in the lobster, shrimp, and bacon. Sauté for 4 minutes. Stir in the rice and glaze for 7 minutes. Add the remaining ingredients and bring to a boil. Remove skillet from heat, pour the mixture in a baking dish, and top with the chicken. Bake in the oven at 350 degrees for 45 minutes.
Serves 6.

CALORIES: 285
PROTEIN: 29.1 gm.
CARBOHYDRATE: 39.6 gm.
FAT: 4.8 gm.

CALCIUM: 63.3 mg.
SODIUM: 687 mg.
CHOLESTEROL: 133 mg.

Vegetables

Belgian Endive

    4 heads Belgian endive
    1 tablespoon diet margarine

¼ cup chicken bouillon
1 tablespoon lemon juice
¼ teaspoon lo-cal sweetener
Dash white pepper

Clean the endive and cut the heads in half lengthwise. In a medium skillet melt the diet margarine. Sauté the endive in the margarine for 3 minutes, turning once. In a small bowl mix the bouillon, lemon juice, lo-cal sweetener, and white pepper. Pour over the vegetables. Cover and braise 10 minutes. Remove the lid from the skillet and continue to cook until the liquid is gone.
Serves 4.

CALORIES: 105.2   CALCIUM: 196 mg.
PROTEIN: 5.9 gm.   SODIUM: 92 mg.
CARBOHYDRATE: 16.6 gm.   CHOLESTEROL: 0 mg.
FAT: 1.6 gm.

Ratatouille

1 eggplant
2 zucchini
2 tablespoons diet margarine
½ cup chopped onion
¼ cup chopped green onion
3 cloves garlic, minced
3 tomatoes, quartered
2 tablespoons minced parsley
⅛ teaspoon black pepper

Cube the eggplant and slice the zucchini. Melt the diet margarine in a saucepan and add the eggplant, zucchini, and remaining ingredients. Cover the pan and continue to cook over low heat for 12 minutes. Pour out into a baking dish and bake 30 minutes in an oven set at 350 degrees.
Serves 4.

CALORIES: 106.9   CALCIUM: 109 mg.
PROTEIN: 4.5 gm.   SODIUM: 9 mg.
CARBOHYDRATE: 16.9 gm.   CHOLESTEROL: 0 mg.
FAT: 3.7 gm.

Braised Celery

12 stalks fresh celery
½ cup water
¼ cup sliced onions
1 carrot, julienne
½ cup chicken bouillon
1 tablespoon diet margarine
Dash pepper

Clean the celery and remove the strings. Cut in half. Place the celery in a saucepan and cover with ½ cup water. Bring to a boil, cover, and turn down the heat to low. Blanch the celery for 5 minutes. Then put the celery in a baking dish and pour over it the onions and carrots. Pour the bouillon over all. Dot with margarine and sprinkle with pepper. Cover with a piece of waxed paper and place in oven. Bake at 375 degrees for 45 minutes.
Serves 4.

CALORIES: 28.6
PROTEIN: .7 gm.
CARBOHYDRATE: 3.3 gm.
FAT: 1.75 gm.

CALCIUM: 12.25 mg.
SODIUM: 280 mg.
CHOLESTEROL: 0 mg.

Cauliflower Melon

1 head cauliflower
2 tablespoons diet margarine
½ teaspoon dry mustard
1 cup cantaloupe balls

Wash and clean the cauliflower and cut into flowerets. Peel the floweret stems. Place the vegetable in a pan of hot water and simmer 8 minutes or until the stems turn yellow green. Remove and cool. Melt the diet margarine in a skillet. Stir in the dry mustard. Toss with the cauliflower and cook for 10 minutes over low heat, stirring frequently. Stir in the melon balls and heat through.
Serves 4.

CALORIES: 62.5
PROTEIN: 3.2 gm.
CARBOHYDRATE: 8.1 gm.
FAT: 3.3 gm.

CALCIUM: 18 mg.
SODIUM: 32.7 mg.
CHOLESTEROL: 0 mg.

Stir-Fry Vegetables

  1 cup cloud ears
  ¹/₄ cup bouillon
  1 cup sliced onions
  1 cup carrots, julienne
  1 teaspoon water
  ¹/₂ cup sliced green onion tops
  1 tablespoon sherry
  1 teaspoon light soy sauce
  2 teaspoons cornstarch

Put the cloud ears into a bowl of water and allow to reconstitute for 30 minutes. When rehydrated, drain. Meanwhile, place the wok over high heat and add the bouillon. When hot, sauté the onions and carrots for 2 minutes, add 1 teaspoon water, and put the lid on the wok for 1 minute. Remove lid. Add the cloud ears and green onion tops. Push the vegetables to the sides of the wok and add the sherry and soy sauce and then stir in the cornstarch. When the sauce thickens and turns clear, add the vegetables and toss. Serve hot.
Serves 4.

CALORIES: 66
PROTEIN: 1.4 gm.
CARBOHYDRATE: 11.4 gm.
FAT: 2.0 gm.

CALCIUM: 33 mg.
SODIUM: 102 mg.
CHOLESTEROL: 0 mg.

Pasta and Rice

White and Wild Rice Croquettes

1 package white and wild rice mix
1 tablespoon diet margarine
1 tablespoon flour
1/4 cup 2 percent milk
1/4 cup water
1 tablespoon sherry
1/4 cup mushrooms, sliced
1 egg, beaten
1 tablespoon water
1/4 cup cracker crumbs

Prepare the white and wild rice mix according to the package directions, but leave out the butter. Meanwhile, prepare the sauce by melting the margarine in a small saucepan. Stir in the flour and cook over medium heat for 4 minutes. Pour in the milk and the 1/4 cup water and whisk until the sauce is smooth and thickened. Stir in the sherry and mushrooms and simmer for 4 minutes over low heat. Cool. Beat the egg with the 1 tablespoon water in a small mixing bowl. In a large mixing bowl place the cooked rice and stir in the sauce. Spread on the bottom of a 9 × 13 baking dish. Chill 1 hour. Cut the rice mixture into 8 equal parts and form into croquettes. Dip in the egg mixture and then in cracker crumbs. Place in a baking dish and bake 25 minutes in an oven set at 325 degrees.

Serves 8.

CALORIES: 144.7   CALCIUM: 15.6 mg.
PROTEIN: 4.8 gm.   SODIUM: 42 mg.
CARBOHYDRATE: 30.6 gm.   CHOLESTEROL: 32 mg.
FAT: 2.3 gm.

Herbed Rice Ring

1 tablespoon diet margarine
1 tablespoon parsley flakes
½ teaspoon thyme
⅛ teaspoon turmeric
Dash white pepper
2 cups chicken bouillon
1 cup uncooked rice
¼ cup chopped green onion tops
Vegetable cooking spray

In a saucepan melt the margarine and pour in the seasonings and bouillon. Bring the liquid to a boil and stir in the rice and green onion tops. Cover and turn the heat down to low. Simmer 25 minutes or until the rice is done. Spray a 4-cup ring mold with vegetable cooking spray and pack the rice in firmly. Unmold quickly onto a serving platter.

Serves 6.

CALORIES: 134.2
PROTEIN: 4.5 gm.
CARBOHYDRATE: 28.3 gm.
FAT: 2.6 gm.

CALCIUM: 43.7 mg.
SODIUM: 273 mg.
CHOLESTEROL: 0 mg.

Pasta Primavera

1 cup parsley leaves
2 cloves garlic, minced
1 onion, coarsely chopped
1 red bell pepper, sliced
1 green bell pepper, sliced
2 zucchini, sliced
3 tomatoes, diced
1 cup broccoli, chopped
2 tablespoons diet margarine
8 ounces tomato juice
2 tablespoons diet catsup
1 teaspoon oregano
1/4 teaspoon pepper
1/2 teaspoon basil
Dash ground cloves
2 cups spaghetti noodles
1 ounce Parmesan cheese

Whirl the parsley leaves with the garlic in a food processor fitted with a steel blade. In a skillet, sauté the onion, red and green peppers, zucchini, tomatoes, and broccoli in the melted diet margarine for 5 minutes. Add the tomato juice, diet catsup, and seasonings and simmer the sauce for 30 minutes. Meanwhile, cook the noodles until they are tender. When done, drain. Pour the sauce over the cooked noodles and sprinkle with Parmesan cheese.
Serves 4.

CALORIES: 136.6
PROTEIN: 6.2 gm.
CARBOHYDRATE: 17.9 gm.
FAT: 3.9 gm.

CALCIUM: 122.6 mg.
SODIUM: 84 mg.
CHOLESTEROL: 11.2

Fish

Baked Bluefish

2 tablespoons diet margarine
1 teaspoon lemon juice
1 clove garlic, minced
1/2 teaspoon Worcestershire sauce
1/8 teaspoon seafood seasoning
2 teaspoons minced parsley
2 teaspoons minced onion
1 teaspoon diet catsup
1/2 teaspoon soy sauce
1/4 cup white wine
4 4-ounce bluefish fillets

In a saucepan, melt the diet margarine. Add the lemon juice, garlic, Worcestershire sauce, seafood seasoning, minced parsley, minced onion, catsup, soy sauce, and white wine. Heat through over medium heat. Brush the wine butter over each of the fillets and place on a baking sheet. Place in an oven set at 350 degrees and bake 25 minutes or until the fish flakes.
Serves 4.

CALORIES: 215
PROTEIN: 30.05 gm.
CARBOHYDRATE: 5.25 gm.
FAT: 12.7 gm.

CALCIUM: 34.38 mg.
SODIUM: 180 mg.
CHOLESTEROL: 84 mg.

Shrimp in a Cream Sauce

1½ pounds shrimp
1½ teaspoons diet margarine
1 tablespoon flour
½ cup 2 percent milk
½ cup white wine
¼ teaspoon white pepper
¼ teaspoon dry mustard
2 ounces Parmesan cheese, grated

In a saucepan, sauté the shrimp in the melted diet margarine 5 minutes or until done. Remove shrimp. Stir the flour into the diet margarine and pour in the milk. Stir until sauce thickens, then add the white wine and seasonings. Return the cooked shrimp to the sauce. Put into ramekins and top with the Parmesan cheese. Place under the broiler until the cheese is melted and browned.
Serves 4.

CALORIES: 262
PROTEIN: 47.6 gm.
CARBOHYDRATE: 6 gm.
FAT: 6.9 gm.

CALCIUM: 402 mg.
SODIUM: 143 mg.
CHOLESTEROL: 294 mg.

Seviche Acapulco

1 pound fillet of sole
3 tablespoons chopped cilantro
2 tomatoes, chopped
½ cup chopped green onion
3 green chilies (not jalapeno), chopped
2 cups lemon juice

Cut the fish into bite-size pieces and place in a mixing bowl. Add the other ingredients to the bowl. Cover. Put in the refrigerator overnight so that fish can "cook."
Serves 4.

CALORIES: 145.4
PROTEIN: 1.7 gm.
CARBOHYDRATE: 14.3 gm.
FAT: .5 gm.

CALCIUM: 28.5 mg.
SODIUM: 203 mg.
CHOLESTEROL: 84 mg.

Cioppino

2 teaspoons diet margarine
1 onion, chopped
1/4 cup chopped green onions
1/4 cup chopped green pepper
1/4 cup chopped parsley
3 cloves garlic, minced
3 tablespoons tomato paste
1 cup rosé wine
2 bay leaves
2 teaspoons seafood seasoning
1/4 teaspoon rosemary
1/4 teaspoon thyme
1/4 teaspoon black pepper
4 whole cloves
2 teaspoons lemon juice
8 ounces tomato juice
1 cup water
8 ounces king crab legs
16 clams in the shells
16 ounces mussels in shells
8 ounces fillet of sole
4 small lobster tails
1 pound shrimp in the shells

Melt the margarine in a large stock pot and add the onions, green onions, green pepper, parsley, garlic, and tomato paste and sauté for 6 minutes. Add the rosé wine, bay leaves, seasonings, and lemon juice. Pour in the tomato juice and add 1 cup of water. Simmer the stew for 1 hour. Add the seafood and cook until just done. Serve in large bowls.
Serves 8.

CALORIES: 207
PROTEIN: 55.2 gm.
CARBOHYDRATE: 14.41 gm.
FAT: 14 gm.

CALCIUM: 186 mg.
SODIUM: 226 mg.
CHOLESTEROL: 405 mg.

Camarones Rancheros

   1½ pounds shrimp
   3 tablespoons chopped Chinese parsley
   4 tomatoes, chopped
   4 green chilies
   4 cloves garlic, minced
   1 cup tomato juice
   1 tablespoon tomato paste
   ½ teaspoon pepper
   1 large onion, chopped

Place all ingredients except the shrimp in a saucepan and bring to a boil. Turn down the heat, cover, and simmer for 25 minutes. Add the shrimp and cook 7 minutes or until the shrimp are done. Serve hot.

Serves 4.

CALORIES: 265
PROTEIN: 44.4 gm.
CARBOHYDRATE: 15.2 gm.
FAT: 2.34 gm.

CALCIUM: 55 mg.
SODIUM: 11 mg.
CHOLESTEROL: 270 mg.

Lobster Crêpes

   1 tablespoon diet margarine
   1½ tablespoons flour
   ½ cup 2 percent milk
   3 tablespoons chopped green onion tops
   1 tablespoon chopped parsley
   2 teaspoons lemon juice
   1 teaspoon grated lemon peel
   ½ cup white wine
   ¼ teaspoon white pepper
   ¼ teaspoon dry mustard
   1 ounce Swiss cheese, grated
   1½ pounds lobster meat
   6 crêpes

Melt the diet margarine in a saucepan and stir in the flour. Cook the roux over medium heat for 3 minutes and stir in the milk. Add the chopped green onion tops and the parsley. Stir in the lemon juice, lemon peel, white wine, pepper, and mustard. Stir in the grated cheese and stir until the sauce is smooth and thick. Add the lobster meat and heat through. Fill the crêpes with the hot lobster mixture and roll up. Place in a casserole dish. Pour the remaining filling over the crêpes and bake for 5 minutes or until hot in an oven set at 350 degrees.

Serves 6.

CALORIES: 164
PROTEIN: 4.1 gm.
CARBOHYDRATE: 4.2 gm.
FAT: 6.7 gm.

CALCIUM: 119.8 mg.
SODIUM: 379 mg.
CHOLESTEROL: 282 mg.

Scallops Annapolis

1 1/2 tablespoons diet margarine
2 tablespoons chopped chives
1/8 teaspoon celery salt
Dash paprika
1/8 teaspoon white pepper
3 tablespoons lime juice
1 1/2 pounds scallops
1 1/2 tablespoons flour
1/4 teaspoon dry mustard
1/2 cup 2 percent milk
1/2 cup white wine
1/4 cup mushrooms, sliced
6 ounces crabmeat, cooked
2 ounces Swiss cheese, grated

In a saucepan, melt the diet margarine and stir in the chives, celery salt, paprika, white pepper, and lime juice. Sauté the scallops until done. Remove scallops from the sauce and set aside. Heat the liquid in the pan over high heat until it just begins to boil. Stir in the flour, add the dry mustard and, using a whisk, pour in the milk and wine. Whisk until smooth and thickened. Stir the cooked scallops and mushrooms into the wine sauce and place in an oval casserole. Top with crabmeat. Sprinkle with grated Swiss cheese. Place under the broiler and broil until the cheese is bubbling and browned. Serve immediately.

Serves 4.

CALORIES: 176
PROTEIN: 26.4 gm.
CARBOHYDRATE: 2.96 gm.
FAT: 4.73 gm.

CALCIUM: 185 mg.
SODIUM: 187 mg.
CHOLESTEROL: 362 mg.

Stuffed Shrimp

4 jumbo shrimp
6 ounces crabmeat
2 tablespoons lime juice
2 tablespoons parsley, chopped
1 tablespoon chopped green onion tops
1 tablespoon diet mayonnaise
1/8 teaspoon seafood seasoning
1 teaspoon prepared mustard
1 egg, beaten
1 tablespoon diet margarine
1 tablespoon flour
1/2 cup 2 percent milk
1/4 cup white wine
1/4 teaspoon white pepper
Vegetable cooking spray
2 ounces Swiss cheese, grated

Clean and shell the shrimp and set aside. Place the crabmeat in a mixing bowl and add the lime juice, parsley, green onion tops, diet mayonnaise, seafood seasoning, prepared mustard, and beaten egg and mix. Chill. Meanwhile, melt the diet margarine in a saucepan and stir in the flour. Cook the roux for 3 minutes over medium heat. Pour in the milk and wine. Cook until smooth and thick. Season with white pepper. Split the jumbo shrimp down the backs without cutting through the shrimp. Stuff the shrimp with the crabmeat. Spray an oval casserole with vegetable cooking spray and spread the bottom with the remaining crabmeat mixture. Top with the stuffed jumbo shrimp and pour the sauce over all. Sprinkle with grated Swiss cheese and place in an oven set at 450 degrees. Bake for 15 minutes or until heated through and the cheese has melted and is slightly browned.
Serves 4.

CALORIES: 168.4
PROTEIN: 15.2 gm.
CARBOHYDRATE: 6.1 gm.
FAT: 8.1 gm.

CALCIUM: 177.4 mg.
SODIUM: 156 mg.
CHOLESTEROL: 200 mg.

Melon-Stuffed Sole

¼ cup chicken bouillon
2 ounces cream cheese
3 ounces Roquefort cheese
3 tablespoons diet mayonnaise
1 tablespoon lemon juice
1 teaspoon anisette
1 tablespoon minced parsley
2 green onions, sliced
⅛ teaspoon hot pepper sauce
⅛ teaspoon Worcestershire sauce
6 ounces raw shrimp
Vegetable cooking spray
8 6-ounce fillets of sole
2 cups cantaloupe balls
1 egg, beaten
1 slice diet bread

Put the chicken bouillon, cream cheese, Roquefort cheese, diet mayonnaise, lemon juice, anisette, parsley, onion, hot pepper sauce, and Worcestershire sauce into a food processor fitted with a steel blade. Whirl until well blended. Cut the shrimp into small pieces. Fold into the cheese mixture. Chill 30 minutes. In a casserole dish that has been sprayed with vegetable spray, layer one-half of the fillets. Top with the cheese-shrimp filling. Spread 1¾ cups cantaloupe balls over this. Reserve ¼ cup for later use. Top with the remaining fillets. Beat the egg until frothy. Baste the fish with the egg. Whirl the bread in a food processor and sprinkle over the fish. Bake 20 minutes or until the fish flakes in an oven set at 375 degrees. Garnish with additional melon balls.
Serves 8.

CALORIES: 250.5   CALCIUM: 67.3 mg.
PROTEIN: 13.1 gm.   SODIUM: 381 mg.
CARBOHYDRATE: 6.8 gm.   CHOLESTEROL: 217 mg.
FAT: 7.8 gm.

Salmon Melon Pâté

2 packets unflavored gelatin
¼ cup water
2 cups rich chicken broth
1 18-ounce can salmon
1 10-ounce package frozen peas
2 cups cantaloupe balls

Dissolve the gelatin in cold water. Heat the chicken broth in a saucepan and stir in the gelatin. Bring to a boil and remove from heat. Cool slightly. In a 1½-quart terrine, put a layer of the gelatin mixture. Refrigerate until set. Meanwhile, clean the salmon, removing all fat, bones, and skin. Put a layer of salmon on top of the gelatin and pour in enough gelatin liquid just to cover the salmon. Chill. When set, put down a layer of peas and cover with the gelatin mixture. Chill. When that is set, top with the melon balls and cover with the remaining gelatin. To serve, cut into slices.
Serves 8.

CALORIES: 137.2
PROTEIN: 16.1 gm.
CARBOHYDRATE: 6.74 gm.
FAT: 39 gm.

CALCIUM: 122.6 mg.
SODIUM: 231 mg.
CHOLESTEROL: 0 mg.

Meats

Veal Cordon Bleu

4 3-ounce veal cutlets, pounded
2 slices Canadian bacon, cut in half
2 ounces sliced Swiss cheese
1 egg, beaten
1 teaspoon water
1 tablespoon 2 percent milk
2 tablespoons flour
2 tablespoons cracker crumbs
White pepper
Dash nutmeg
2 tablespoons diet margarine

Cut each cutlet in half and pound very thin. Place 1 slice of Canadian bacon and 1 slice of Swiss cheese on half the veal cutlets.

Top with the remaining 4 cutlets. In a mixing bowl, beat the egg with the water and milk. Sprinkle the cutlet packages with flour, then brush with the egg and sprinkle with the cracker crumbs. Dust with pepper and nutmeg. Melt the margarine and drizzle over the cutlets. Bake for 25 minutes or until done in an oven set at 400 degrees.
Serves 4.

CALORIES: 340.6
PROTEIN: 12.1 gm.
CARBOHYDRATE: 4.1 gm.
FAT: 20.4 gm.

CALCIUM: 36 mg.
SODIUM: 475 mg.
CHOLESTEROL: 155 mg.

Veal Parmesan

1½ pounds veal cutlets
2 tablespoons flour
2 ounces Parmesan cheese
2 tablespoons diet margarine
Vegetable cooking spray
1 cup tomato juice
1 tablespoon diet catsup
¼ cup minced onion
2 tablespoons Chinese parsley, chopped
¼ teaspoon pepper
2 teaspoons minced green pepper
3 cloves garlic
1 ounce Parmesan cheese

Pound the cutlets very thin. Mix the flour and one ounce of the grated Parmesan cheese and dredge cutlets. Melt the diet margarine in a skillet that has been sprayed with vegetable cooking spray. Brown the cutlets on both sides. Meanwhile, make a sauce with the remaining ingredients except for the remaining 1 ounce of Parmesan cheese. Cook the sauce over high heat, stirring frequently. Reduce the sauce to ½ cup. Place cutlets in a baking dish and top with the sauce. Sprinkle with cheese. Bake for 10 minutes or until the cheese has melted in an oven set at 450 degrees.
Serves 4.

CALORIES: 330.4
PROTEIN: 31.7 gm.
CARBOHYDRATE: 7.3 gm.
FAT: 18.4 gm.

CALCIUM: 181.6 mg.
SODIUM: 296 mg.
CHOLESTEROL: 185 mg.

Poultry

Chicken Pâté

1 teaspoon unflavored gelatin
¼ cup dry white wine
8 ounces ground veal
8 ounces ground chicken breast
1 ounce pork fat
2 eggs, beaten
1 tablespoon chopped chives
¼ teaspoon white pepper
¼ teaspoon thyme leaves
1 ounce Cognac
4 strips bacon
1 boneless chicken breast

Dissolve the gelatin in the wine and put in a small saucepan and bring to a boil. Remove from heat. Meanwhile, in a mixing bowl combine the veal, ground chicken breast, pork fat, eggs, chives, spices, and Cognac. Put into a food processor fitted with a steel blade. Whirl until the ingredients are smooth and fine. Put 2 of the bacon strips in the bottom of a loaf pan. Then put ½ of the meat mixture on top of that. Cut the chicken breast into thin strips and put on the loaf lengthwise. Top with the remaining pâté mix. Put the 2 remaining strips of bacon on the pâté. Cover with foil and puncture a hole in the foil. Put the loaf pan in a large baking dish with 1 inch of water. Bake in an oven set at 350 degrees for 1½ hours. Meanwhile, cover a brick with foil. Remove pâté from oven. Remove lid and put the brick on top of the pâté. Cool. Refrigerate several days before serving. Cut into 12 slices.
Makes 12 servings.

CALORIES: 94.4
PROTEIN: 11.1 gm.
CARBOHYDRATE: 3 gm.
FAT: 5.3 gm.

CALCIUM: 8.1 mg.
SODIUM: 43 mg.
CHOLESTEROL: 95 mg.

Desserts

Cherry Cheesecake
    1 cup crushed zwieback
    2 tablespoons diet margarine, melted
    1/2 teaspoon lo-cal sweetener
    1 tablespoon unflavored gelatin
    1/4 cup water
    2 egg yolks, beaten
    1/2 cup 2 percent milk
    1/3 cup ricotta cheese
    1/2 teaspoon lo-cal sweetener
    1/2 teaspoon cherry extract
    1 1/2 teaspoons vanilla
    1 ounce kirsch
    1/3 cup water
    4 egg whites
    1/2 cup whipped dessert topping
    1 cup canned pitted cherries
    1/2 teaspoon lo-cal sweetener

Place the zwieback in a mixing bowl and, using a pastry fork, blend in the melted diet margarine. Add 1/2 teaspoon lo-cal sweetener. Remove 2 tablespoons of the crumb mix and reserve for later use. Press the crumb crust into the bottom and sides of an 8-inch springform pan. Chill in the refrigerator. Meantime, place the gelatin in a small bowl and pour the 1/4 cup water over to dissolve. In a small saucepan, put the egg yolks, milk, ricotta cheese, lo-cal sweetener, cherry extract, vanilla, and kirsch. Add 1/3 cup water and place over medium heat. Stir in the dissolved gelatin. Stir constantly for 20 minutes. When the sauce coats a spoon, remove from the heat and chill 15 minutes or until the sauce just begins to thicken. Meanwhile, beat the egg whites until they form stiff peaks. Fold the egg whites into the custard mixture and then fold in the whipped dessert topping. Pour the filling into the springform pan. Cover and place in the refrigerator for 6 hours or until it is firm. Top with the cherries sweetened with 1/2 teaspoon lo-cal sweetener and sprinkle with the 2 tablespoons of reserved crumb mixture.
Serves 10.

CALORIES: 131.3   CALCIUM: 34 mg.
PROTEIN: 6.1 gm.   SODIUM: 59.2 mg.
CARBOHYDRATE: 14.8 gm.   CHOLESTEROL: 1.2 mg.
FAT: 4.2 gm.

Mocha Mousse

    1 tablespoon instant coffee granules
    1 ounce brandy
    3 tablespoons hot water
    1 recipe Soufflé Base

Dissolve the coffee in the hot water and stir in the brandy. Make 1 recipe Soufflé Base according to the directions on page 164 and stir in the coffee mixture. Cool. Fold into the whipped egg whites. Chill in a soufflé dish.
Serves 6.

CALORIES: 92.6
PROTEIN: 9.5 gm.
CARBOHYDRATE: 3.4 gm.
FAT: 3.7 gm.

CALCIUM: 58.4 mg.
SODIUM: 136.1 mg.
CHOLESTEROL: 46.1 mg.

Crêpes Melon Suzette

    1 recipe Crêpes
    2 oranges
    Peel from 2 oranges
    Peel from 1 lemon
    1 tablespoon orange blossom water
    1 ounce orange liqueur
    ½ cup orange juice
    3 tablespoons lemon juice
    ¾ teaspoon lo-cal sweetener
    2 teaspoons vanilla
    1 ounce kirsch
    1 tablespoon Maraschino
    1 ounce rum
    1 cup watermelon balls

Prepare the crêpes according to the directions on page 186 and set aside 4. Freeze the remaining 12 between sheets of waxed paper for later use. Peel 2 oranges and juice them. Grate the peel from both oranges. Grate the peel from the lemon and juice it. In a saucepan, prepare the sauce: Combine all the ingredients except the rum and the watermelon balls and place over low heat. Simmer 30 minutes. When ready to serve, fold the crêpes into fourths. Place the crêpes in a pan and pour the sauce over them. Heat through, turning the crêpes once. Pour in the rum and flame. When the flames go out, stir in the melon balls. Heat through. Allow 1 crêpe per person. *Serves 4.*

CALORIES: 119.5　　　　CALCIUM: 49.4 mg.
PROTEIN: 2.4 gm.　　　　SODIUM: 110.7 mg.
CARBOHYDRATE: 17.4 gm.　CHOLESTEROL: 0 mg.
FAT: 1 gm.

Fudge Mousse in Melon

    2 ounces sweet chocolate
    2 tablespoons diet margarine
    3 packets lo-cal sweetener
    1 tablespoon hot water
    1 teaspoon instant coffee
    1 tablespoon brandy
    1 whole egg
    ¼ cup diet whipped topping
    6 egg whites
    1 cantaloupe
    Fresh mint sprigs

In the top of a double boiler, melt the chocolate, diet margarine, and 2 packets of the lo-cal sweetener. Stir in the hot water and instant coffee and brandy. Beat the egg slightly and then stir into the chocolate mixture. Cool the chocolate over ice. Meanwhile, beat the diet whipped topping until it is stiff. While beating the egg whites, pour in the remaining packet of lo-cal sweetener. Continue beating until the egg whites form stiff peaks. Carefully fold the whipped topping and egg whites into the chocolate mixture. Pour into serving dishes and refrigerate overnight. To serve, cut the cantaloupe into 6 pieces, put fudge mousse on top of each slice. Garnish with sprigs of fresh mint.
Serves 6.

CALORIES: 53.6　　　　CALCIUM: 10.6 mg.
PROTEIN: 4.6 gm.　　　　SODIUM: 70.1 mg.
CARBOHYDRATE: 1.5 gm.　CHOLESTEROL: 42.1 mg.
FAT: 3.5 gm.

Lemon Melon Mousse

1 recipe Soufflé Base
2 teaspoons lemon extract
2 teaspoons grated lemon peel
1 cup Casaba melon balls

Make 1 recipe Soufflé Base according to the directions on page 164 and add the lemon extract and grated lemon peel. Fold in the egg whites from the Soufflé Base and the melon balls. Pour into a soufflé dish. Chill.
Serves 6.

CALORIES: 93
PROTEIN: 9.8 gm.
CARBOHYDRATE: 4.9 gm.
FAT: 3.7 gm.

CALCIUM: 61.2 mg.
SODIUM: 138.3 mg.
CHOLESTEROL: 34.6 mg.

Peach Melon Chiffon

2 envelopes unflavored gelatin
1½ cups tangerine juice
2 eggs, separated
1 tablespoon cornstarch
4 packets lo-cal sweetener
Salt
3 cups low-fat cottage cheese
1 teaspoon vanilla
1 cup chopped peaches
¼ cup graham cracker crumbs

Dissolve the gelatin in ½ cup tangerine juice. Separate the eggs. Put the cornstarch and the remaining tangerine juice in a saucepan. Bring to a boil and cook until it thickens. Put the dissolved gelatin in a blender and add the egg yolks, lo-cal sweetener, salt, cottage cheese, and vanilla. Blend until smooth. Stir in the peaches. Chill at least ½ hour or until it begins to set. Beat the egg whites until stiff. Fold into the peach mixture. Pour into an 8-inch springform pan and sprinkle the top with cracker crumbs. Chill. To serve, remove from springform pan.
Serves 16.

CALORIES: 108.8
PROTEIN: 1.1 gm.
CARBOHYDRATE: 26.2 gm.
FAT: .3 gm.

CALCIUM: 24.4 mg.
SODIUM: 107.6 mg.
CHOLESTEROL: 35.3 mg.

Poached Pears with Melon Sauce

  4 packets lo-cal sweetener
  2 cups red wine
  1/4 cup apple juice
  2 tablespoons water
  1/8 teaspoon grated lemon peel
  2 teaspoons lemon juice
  1 whole clove
  Pinch allspice
  1 2-inch cinnamon stick
  1 cup puree of cantaloupe
  4 pears
  1 teaspoon gelatin

In a small saucepan that will just hold the pears, put the lo-cal sweetener, wine, apple juice, water, lemon peel, lemon juice, spices, and cantaloupe puree. Bring the syrup to a boil for 5 minutes. Cool. Peel the pears carefully, leaving on the stems for decoration. Trim the pears on the bottom so that they will not fall over in the pan. Pour the wine syrup over the pears in the saucepan, covering them. Cover the pan and simmer over low heat for 35 minutes or until the pears are tender. Remove pears from syrup and place in an oval dish. Dissolve the gelatin in the saucepan with the syrup and bring to a boil for 5 minutes or until the syrup is reduced by half. Place in the refrigerator and chill for 1 hour. Spoon the slightly thickened syrup over the pears. Chill.
Serves 4.

CALORIES: 140.5   CALCIUM: 14.2 mg.
PROTEIN: 1.9 gm.   SODIUM: 11 mg.
CARBOHYDRATE: 41.3 gm. CHOLESTEROL: 0 mg.
FAT: 15.7 gm.

Watermelon Ice

½ cup puree of watermelon
¼ teaspoon lemon juice
2 cups water
4 packets lo-cal sweetener
1½ tablespoons unflavored gelatin
¼ cup cold water

Put the watermelon puree, lemon juice, 2 cups water, and sweetener in a saucepan and bring to a boil. Dissolve the gelatin in ¼ cup cold water. Stir into the boiling liquid. Pour into a shallow pan and freeze. When frozen remove and whirl in a food processor fitted with a steel blade. Return to the pan and refreeze. Repeat this process twice more. To serve, remove from freezer 20 minutes before serving and put in the refrigerator.
Serves 6.

CALORIES: 14
PROTEIN: 2.1 gm.
CARBOHYDRATE: .8 gm.
FAT: Trace

CALCIUM: 1.7 mg.
SODIUM: .3 mg.
CHOLESTEROL: 0 mg.

22

Quick, Easy Exercises

This diet is not coupled with a rigorous exercise program. The midshipmen in our diet plan were sent to us for a healthy diet only. The exercise program available to all midshipmen comes from Red Romo, head trainer of the Athletic Department. The Naval Academy has almost every sport and one of the most outstanding athletic departments in the country. Captain Bo Coppage, USN (Retired), sees to it that his midshipmen have the best educators, facilities, and equipment available. The plebes rise around 5:30 A.M. and are required to do calisthenics or jog a prescribed distance before their 6:30 A.M. breakfast is served. The daily athletic period begins at 3:00 P.M. every day, and exercise frequently includes running the "wall": The Naval Academy sits on the Chesapeake Bay at the mouth of the Severn River and a sea wall surrounds much of the grounds. Sometimes this 5-mile run is assigned as punishment, but most of the time it is done for fun and recreation.

I asked Red Romo to give the dieters some specific exercises that would work on the parts of the body most prone to collecting fat. I also asked him to give us his theory on keeping in shape for those of us past college age. If you already exercise add these exercises to your list. They will take you about 15 minutes of your day, and after the first two days you will feel great. Be sure not to overdo. You do not want to hurt yourself or pull any of those long-unused muscles. If you do these as soon as you wake up—and *always* before breakfast—you won't have to worry about exercising for the rest of the day.

While you are going through these exercises, remember that Red Romo has trained many famous star athletes. One who comes quickly to mind is Roger Staubach. Here are Red's exercises and suggestions:

"If you are wondering whether you should do exercises or not, here are some guidelines: Those working in an office should, during their working hours, move around every hour so as to be not sitting for long periods of time."

He also recommends taking a half-hour walk every day after dinner. Dress comfortably and walk with someone at a nice easy pace. In other words, keep those bones and muscles moving!

Now here are some specific exercises.

Red Romo's Exercises to Keep in Shape

Exercise A

Hide your knife and fork.

Exercise B

Push away from the table.

Exercise C

Eat slowly. Do not fill up on liquids. It is important to eat salads, vegetables, fish, and meat but not in large portions. If you feel hungry between meals, then have a bowl of fruit handy—apples, pears, grapes, etc. Stay away from those fast food restaurants or fancy French places (and note that Red Romo is also in the restaurant business. His cozy little restaurant tucked behind the Capitol building on State Circle is a frequent haunt of the midshipmen). Seriously, here are seven of the best exercises to keep you in shape.

Exercise One: Stomach Exercise

While standing or talking to someone, tighten your stomach muscles and hold for ten seconds at a time. Do this during the entire conversation. This can also be done while you are driving your car.

Exercise Two: Sit-Ups

Work alone or with a partner: Start with ten sit-ups. As with all exercises, do at a slow, easy pace. If you are doing your sit-ups with a partner, have the partner hold your feet while you do the sit-ups. Keep your hands behind your head. Increase by five sit-ups per day until you are up to 120.

Exercise Three: Touching Toes

Bending from the waist with your arms outstretched, touch your toes or go down as far as possible. Do these for thirty seconds and increase the time by fifteen seconds every day until you do them for three minutes.

Exercise Four: Sitting Position

Spread your legs apart and be sure they are straight. Reach out and touch your toes with the alternate arm. Stretch as far as you can and do not bend the knees.

Exercise Five: Trunk Rotation

Put your hands on your hips and your feet about a foot apart. Stand up straight and look straight ahead. Rotate first to the left and then to the right. At the beginning, do for thirty seconds per day. Increase this by thirty seconds each day until you reach four minutes.

Exercise Six: Broom Handle

Use a broom handle as if it were a weight bar. In the standing position use the handle as if you were pressing overhead and down. Do three sets of eight; repeat. Rest thirty seconds between each set.

Exercise Seven: Rowing

This exercise strengthens the abdominal muscles and also exercises the leg extensors and flexor muscles. Start slow to moderate.

Starting position: Lie flat on your back, with your arms extended over the head. Put the feet together.

Movement: Sit up and at the same time bend the knees sharply. Lean forward, swinging the arms forward to a rowing position with the knees together and against the chest, feet flat on the ground, heels close to the buttocks, and arms extended forward. Return to starting position. Do this ten times to start and increase by as many as you can.

Extra Exercises

If possible, swim or ride a bicycle each day. Or do the Side Straddle Hop (the same as jumping jacks). The midshipmen do 150 side straddle hops a day or more. You could start with fifty and increase after that.

Index